This concise practical guide deals with the investigations, diagnosis and treatment of all the common metabolic bone diseases and disorders of calcium metabolism. Osteoporosis, osteomalacia, Paget's disease, hyperaemia and hypocalcaemia are all covered, and the volume concludes ith a brief look at some of the rarer conditions which might occasionally be encountered. Each chapter summarises the most recent advances in the understanding of the aetiology of these diseases and provides practical guidance on new and established treatment regimes. The volume will be a valuable source of guidance for the many physicians, based in hospitals and general practice, who encounter patients with these diseases.

The volume will appeal broadly to consultants and senior registrars in general medicine, geriatric medicine, rheumatology, endocrinology, orthopaedic surgery and to general practitioners.

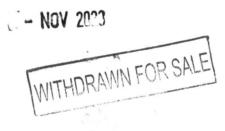

THE MANAGEMENT OF COMMON METABOLIC
BONE DISORDERS

THE MANAGEMENT OF COMMON METABOLIC BONE DISORDERS

GORDON CAMPBELL, JULIET COMPSTON AND
ADRIAN CRISP

Addenbrooke's Hospital, Cambridge

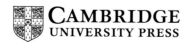

CAMBRIDGE
UNIVERSITY PRESS

Published by the Press Syndicate of the University of Cambridge
The Pitt Building, Trumpington Street, Cambridge CB2 1RP
40 West 20th Street, New York, NY 10011-4211, USA
10 Stamford Road, Oakleigh, Melbourne 3166, Australia

First published 1993

Printed in Great Britain at the University Press, Cambridge

A catalogue record for this book is available from the British Library

Library of Congress cataloguing in publication data
Campbell, Gordon, MRCP.
The management of common metabolic bone disorders / Gordon
Campbell, Juliet Compston, and Adrian Crisp.
p. cm.
Includes index.
ISBN 0–521–43037–2 (hardback). – ISBN 0–521–43623–0 (pbk.)
1. Bones – Metabolism – Disorders – Handbooks, manuals, etc.
I. Compston, Juliet. II. Crips, Adrian. III. Title.
[DNLM: 1. Bone Diseases, Metabolic. WE 250 C187m 1994]
RC930.C27 1994
616.7'16 – dc20 93–10390 CIP

ISBN 0 521 43037 2 hardback
ISBN 0 521 43623 0 paperback

VN

Contents

Preface

The increasing interest in metabolic bone disease over the past few years is well illustrated by the increase in the number of references cited for osteoporosis in *Index Medicus* over the last 5 years, there being over 450 for 1991 alone. Increasingly, it is being appreciated that osteoporosis is not inevitable, that prevention is certainly achievable, and that treatment regimes which reduce fracture rates do exist for established disease. Thus interest is no longer confined to endocrinologists with a special interest in metabolic bone disease, but to a much wider medical field, including general physicians, geriatricians, gynaecologists, orthopaedic surgeons, primary care physicians and rheumatologists, amongst others. Public, as well as general medical, awareness of these diseases, especially osteoporosis, has also grown. Much progress has also been made in our understanding of other metabolic bone disorders, e.g. osteogenesis imperfecta.

The aim of this book is to provide an update on the investigation and treatment of the major metabolic bone diseases in order to help non-specialists, both in hospital and general practice, who may not have access to a bone clinic. Some of the rarer disorders are also discussed in order to provide hopefully useful background information which, in addition, should be of help to those revising for post-graduate qualifications.

1

The pathogenesis and investigation of metabolic bone disease

The physiology and biochemistry of bone

Bone composition and structure

The adult skeleton contains 99% of the total body calcium. It serves three main functions: first, it has an important mechanical function and serves as a site for the attachment of muscles, secondly, it protects vital organs and accommodates the bone marrow, and thirdly it serves an important metabolic function, providing a huge reservoir of calcium and phosphate ions. Bone is a connective tissue composed of an extracellular collagenous matrix (Type 1 collagen) and a ground substance containing glycosaminoglycans. Within, and on, this matrix are crystals of hydroxyapatite which provide the mineralised phase of bone. In adult bone, the collagen fibres show a preferential orientation, resulting in a lamellar appearance (Fig. 1.1); these lamellae generally run parallel to one another in trabecular bone and are arranged in concentric rings in cortical bone. Woven bone is characterised by randomly orientated collagen fibres and occurs in growing bone and in disease states characterised by increased bone turnover.

Non-collagenous proteins comprise 10–15% of total bone protein and include cell attachment proteins such as fibronectin, thrombospondin, osteopontin and bone sialoprotein, glycosaminoglycans, gamma-carboxylated (gla) proteins, notably osteocalcin and growth factors, for example, bone morphogenetic proteins and insulin-like growth factors. The functions of these proteins are poorly understood but include osteoclast attachment to mineralised bone matrix, collagen fibrillogenesis, mineralisation of bone matrix and regulation of bone remodelling. The bone morphogenetic proteins include most of the family of transforming growth factor proteins and possess the ability to stimulate bone formation in vivo.

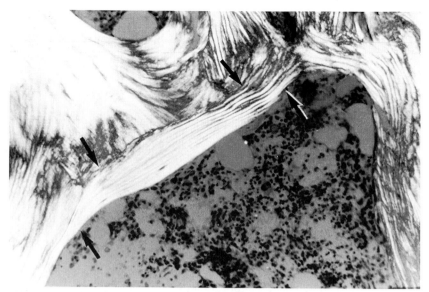

Fig. 1.1. Section of iliac crest trabecular bone viewed under polarised light to show lamellar bone in a bone structural unit (arrowed). (Reproduced with permission of *British Medical Bulletin*, 1992, **48**, 309–44.)

At the macroscopic level, there are two major forms of bone, cortical or compact and trabecular or spongy. Cortical bone comprises approximately 80% of the skeleton and is found mainly in the shafts of long bones and on the surface of flat bones, whilst trabecular bone occurs at the ends of long bones and inside the cortical shell of flat bones. Structurally, cortical bone is composed of compact bone concentrically arranged around central canals containing blood vessels, lymphatics, nerves and connective tissue (Haversian system); the Haversian systems are in communication with one another by means of transverse canals (Volkmann's canals). Trabecular bone structure varies in different parts of the skeleton but essentially consists of interconnecting plates and bars which are continuous with the inner side of the cortex and within which lies haematopoietic or fatty marrow (Fig. 1.2). Trabecular bone has a much higher surface to volume ratio than cortical bone, and hence considerably greater potential for metabolic activity.

Bone surfaces and cells

There are two main bone surfaces, where the bone is in contact with soft tissues: the external periosteal surface and the inner endosteal surface.

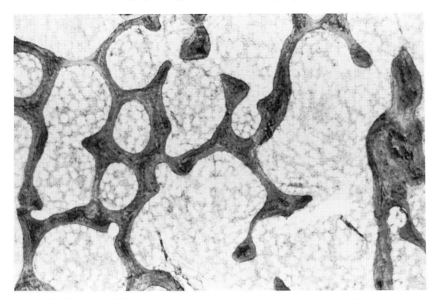

Fig. 1.2. Section of iliac crest trabecular bone to show interconnecting structure.

Bone remodelling takes place on these surfaces, which in the quiescent state are covered by a thin collagenous membrane which itself is covered by a continuous layer of flat lining cells. There are three main cell types associated with bone, namely osteoblasts, osteoclasts and osteocytes. However, it is recognised increasingly that other cells, present in the bone marrow, also have profound effects upon bone remodelling.

Osteoblasts are derived from bone marrow stromal stem cells, and are responsible for the synthesis of bone matrix and its subsequent mineralisation. During bone formation they appear plump and are seen lined up along the newly forming matrix; after bone formation has been completed they may become buried within calcified bone, where they become osteocytes, or may change to become flattened cells which lie on quiescent bone surfaces.

Osteoclasts are large, multinucleated cells which resorb bone (Fig. 1.3) and are derived from haematopoietic cells, probably from the macrophage/monocyte lineage. In normal bone they are far fewer in number than osteoblasts and are generally seen in association with resorption cavities. When examined by electron microscopy, a characteristic ruffled border can be seen; this plays an important role in the process of resorption.

Osteocytes are small, flattened cells which form part of an extensive bone canalicular network by which the calcified bone matrix communicates with

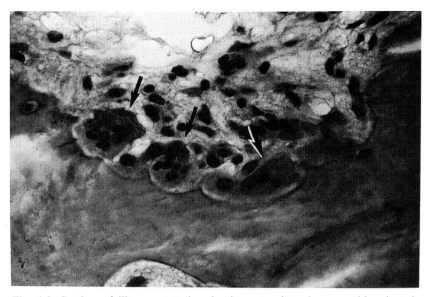

Fig. 1.3. Section of iliac crest trabecular bone to show large, multinucleated osteoclasts (arrowed) and resorption of mineralised bone.

the bone surface via the lining cells (Fig. 1.4); this network also contains the bone extra-cellular fluid (ECF) which is separated from the systemic ECF by the lining cells covering the bone surface. In lamellar bone, osteocytes are arranged parallel to the axis of the collagen fibres whereas, in woven bone, they are larger and show a much more haphazard distribution. In cortical bone, osteocytes are arranged circumferentially around the concentric bone lamellae.

Bone remodelling

The process of bone remodelling is a surface event which serves to replace old bone with new, mechanically more competent bone. It occurs mainly on the endosteal surface of bone, i.e. at the interface of bone and marrow; in the normal adult skeleton, approximately 20% of the trabecular bone surface is undergoing remodelling at any one time. In trabecular bone, the process occurs at discrete sites described as bone remodelling units and essentially consists of the removal of a quantum of bone, by osteoclasts, followed by formation of a similar amount of bone, by osteoblasts, in the cavity so formed (Fig. 1.5). The sequence of events is always that of resorption followed by formation (coupling) and, in the young adult

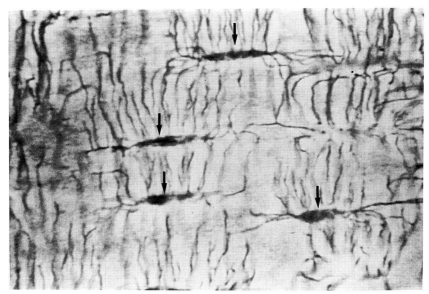

Fig. 1.4. Osteocytes (arrowed) and the canalicular network.

skeleton, the amount of bone resorbed and formed within individual units is quantitatively similar (balance). Bone loss may result from one or both of two processes. In the first, termed remodelling imbalance, the amount of bone formed within individual units relative to that resorbed is reduced, owing to decreased formation, increased resorption or both (Fig. 1.6(*a*)). The other mechanism for bone loss at this level is increased activation of new remodelling units (increased activation frequency), which may lead to rapid bone loss, particularly if combined with remodelling imbalance (Fig. 1.6(*b*)). Conditions characterised by increased activation frequency are described as high turnover bone disease.

The initial stage in the remodelling process is activation, in which a previously quiescent bone surface is 'prepared' for resorption. This involves retraction of lining cells and digestion of the thin collagenous membrane covering the bone surface. Osteoclast precursors are then recruited to the site, and undergo fusion to form mature osteoclasts. These osteoclasts become attached to the mineralised bone surface, a process involving glycoprotein receptors known as integrins, and subsequently produce an acidic environment in which bone mineral is dissolved and collagen digested. The completion of resorption is followed by the reversal phase, during which the cement line is laid down at the base of the resorption cavity and is characterised by the presence of mononuclear cells

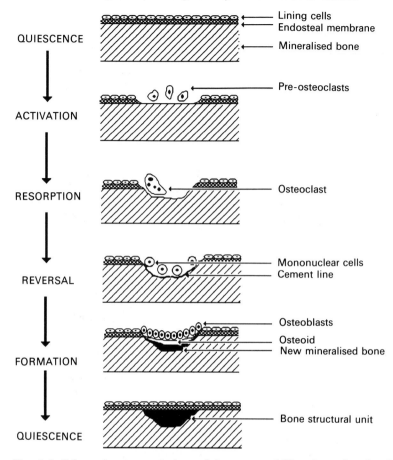

QUIESCENCE ⟶ Lining cells
Endosteal membrane
Mineralised bone

ACTIVATION ⟶ Pre-osteoclasts

RESORPTION ⟶ Osteoclast

REVERSAL ⟶ Mononuclear cells
Cement line

FORMATION ⟶ Osteoblasts
Osteoid
New mineralised bone

QUIESCENCE ⟶ Bone structural unit

Fig. 1.5. Schematic representation of bone remodelling in trabecular bone. (Reproduced with permission from *British Medical Bulletin*, 1992, **48**, 309–44, redrawn from Parfitt, A. M., *Calcif Tissue Int.* 1974, **36**, S37–S45.)

in the cavity. Bone formation occurs in two stages: the formation of osteoid, or unmineralised bone, followed by its mineralisation. Collagen matrix is secreted by osteoblasts in the cavity to form an osteoid seam; following a period of osteoid maturation, mineralisation of the matrix proceeds. The osteoid maturation period averaged over the entire bone surface is known as the mineralisation lag time. When bone formation has been completed, the unit becomes known as a bone structural unit (Fig. 1.1); these newly formed packets of bone continue to increase in mineral density but the overlying surface returns to its former state of quiescence.

In the normal adult skeleton, the process of bone remodelling within an individual unit takes between four and seven months to be completed.

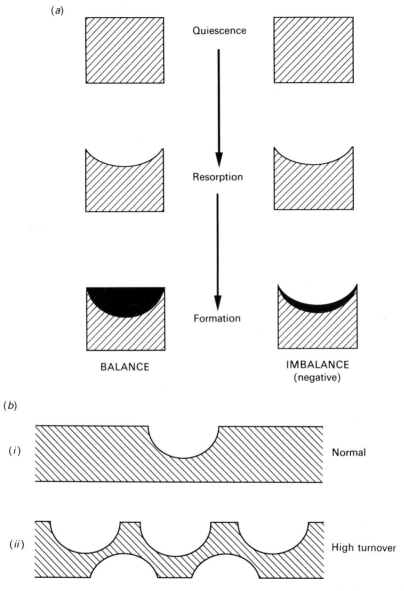

Fig. 1.6. Mechanism of bone loss: (*a*) remodelling imbalance, (*b*) increased activation frequency.

Table. 1.1. *Effect of systemic hormones on bone*

Hormone	Effects
Parathyroid hormone	Increased resorption/turnover
	Anabolic effect (intermittent dosage)
1,25-dihydroxyvitamin D_3	Increased resorption
	Correction of mineralisation defect in rickets/osteomalacia
	Decreased turnover
Calcitonin	Decreased resorption/turnover
Thyroxine	Increased turnover
Oestrogen	Decreased resorption/turnover
	?anabolic effect
Androgens	Decreased resorption/turnover
	?anabolic effect
Growth hormone	Decreased resorption/turnover
	?anabolic effect
Glucocorticoids	Increased resorption/turnover (acute effect)
	Reduced formation

Most of this time is occupied by formation, resorption and reversal accounting for only 36 weeks.

Control of bone remodelling

Mechanical, systemic hormonal and local factors are all involved in the regulation of bone remodelling. Mechanical stresses may be transmitted via the osteocytic/canalicular network to the lining cells, which then respond by releasing factors which initiate activation of bone remodelling. The effect of systemic hormones on bone remodelling may be mediated by the release of local factors; for example, both parathyroid hormone and growth hormone are known to stimulate the production of insulin-like growth factors. Local factors affect bone remodelling mainly via effects on the differentiation and proliferation of bone cells; they are produced by bone cells, bone matrix and cells in the bone microenvironment and act in a paracrine or autocrine manner. They may also be responsible for the regulation of many aspects of osteoclastic function by osteoblasts, and for the coupling of bone formation to resorption during the process of remodelling.

Systemic hormones

Systemic hormones affecting bone remodelling are shown in Table 1.1. Many of these have multiple effects which may be related to dose or mode

Table. 1.2. *Some local factors which affect bone remodelling*

Interleukins 1 + 6	IL-1, IL-6
Tumour necrosis factor alpha + beta	TNFα, TNFβ
Insulin-like growth factor 1 + 2	IGF-1, IGF-2
Transforming growth factors alpha + beta	TGFα, TGFβ
Platelet derived growth factors	PDGF
Fibroblast growth factors	FGF
Beta₂microglobulin	β2μM
Macrophage colony stimulating factor	M-CSF
Granulocyte macrophage colony stimulating factor	GM-CSF
Parathyroid hormone related peptide	PTH-RP
Epidermal growth factor	EGF
Interferon gamma	IFNγ
Prostaglandins	PGs
Bone morphogenetic proteins (e.g. osteogenin, osteoinductive factor)	BMPs
Vasoactive intestinal peptide	VIP
Calcitonin gene-related peptide	CGRP
Leukaemia inhibitory factor	LIF

of administration. Thus parathyroid hormone stimulates bone resorption and inhibits bone formation in vitro; in vivo, however, intermittent dosage produces significant anabolic effects. Glucocorticoids stimulate bone resorption indirectly by reducing intestinal calcium absorption and thus increasing secretion of parathyroid hormone. Short-term administration stimulates bone formation, whilst long-term use leads to reduced bone formation owing to a decrease in the replication of osteoblastic cells. The active metabolite of vitamin D, 1,25-dihydroxyvitamin D, stimulates bone resorption and inhibits bone formation in vitro; in vivo, however, it stimulates the production of osteocalcin from osteoblasts, indicating that, under some circumstances, it may stimulate bone formation. Sex steroids are important physiological regulators of bone mass, and oestrogen receptors have been demonstrated on osteoblast-like cells, although their physiological function is uncertain. There is some evidence that oestrogens affect bone mass by altering the production of cytokines from bone cells and cells in the bone microenvironment.

Local factors (Table 1.2)

A large number of cytokines and growth factors have been identified which are produced by bone cells and cells in the bone marrow and which affect bone cells and remodelling in vitro. There is increasing evidence that these local factors are important regulators of bone remodelling in vivo, possibly acting as mediators for systemic hormones and mechanical stimuli. Some factors, for example interleukin 1(IL-1) and tumour necrosis factor (TNF), stimulate bone resorption; the effect of TNF may be at least partly mediated via IL-1 production. Others, such as transforming growth factors (TGFs) and insulin-like growth factors (IGFs) have predominantly anabolic effects on bone. However, the actions of many factors differ according to the experimental conditions used and in vivo they are likely to be complex and interactive. Some factors are important in the pathogenesis of hypercalcaemia associated with malignancy. Thus parathyroid hormone-related peptide (PTH-rp) is responsible for hypercalcaemia in some cases of humoral hypercalcaemia of malignancy and IL-1 and TNF play an important role in hypercalcaemia associated with myelomatosis.

Calcium and phosphorus homeostasis and metabolism

The adult human contains approximately 1000 grams of calcium, of which 99% is in bone. Calcium homeostasis is tightly regulated by the effects of parathyroid hormone and 1,25-dihydroxyvitamin D on intestinal calcium absorption, renal tubular reabsorption and bone resorption (Fig. 1.7). The dietary intake of calcium varies considerably, and effective intake depends on a variety of factors including the source of calcium, efficiency of intestinal absorption and interaction with other nutrients. Dietary intake in the UK is generally between 500 and 1000 mg daily, of which 15–70% may be absorbed from the intestine. There is a considerable capacity to adapt to low calcium intakes by increasing intestinal absorption, although this adaptive response shows considerable variance. Absorptive efficiency decreases with age and in association with oestrogen deficiency at the menopause. Between five and seven grams of calcium are filtered daily by the kidney, with reabsorption of all but about 250 mg. The daily blood/bone exchange of calcium is approximately 500 mg. Approximately 500 mg are excreted daily in the faeces and there is also a small obligatory loss of calcium from the skin.

90% of total body phosphorus is found in the skeleton and serum concentrations are less tightly regulated than in the case of calcium, changes in dietary intake being responsible for much of the variation. Phosphorus homeostasis is preserved largely through control of its renal conservation, which, in turn, is regulated by parathyroid hormone.

Parathyroid hormone

Parathyroid hormone secretion is predominantly controlled by the concentration of ionised calcium in the extracellular fluid, hypocalcaemia

Diet 500–1000 mg/day

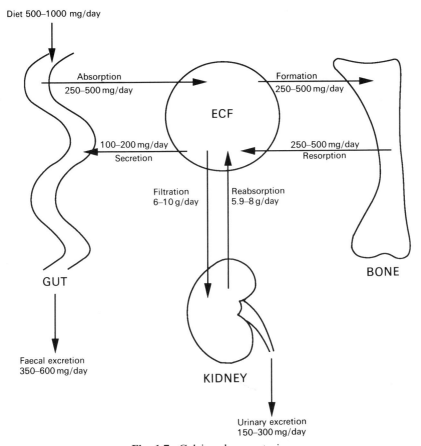

Fig. 1.7. Calcium homeostasis.

stimulating its secretion and hypercalcaemia suppressing it. The intact hormone, which contains 84 amino acids, is rapidly cleared from the circulation with a half-life of less than four minutes. Circulating parathyroid hormone is heterogeneous and consists mainly of inactive C-terminal fragments.

The major function of parathyroid hormone is to maintain calcium and phosphate homeostasis, an effect achieved by actions on the bone, renal tubule and the renal 1 alpha-hydroxylase system. It has complex effects on bone, increased bone resorption occurring with chronically raised serum levels but anabolic effects being seen with intermittent administration of relatively low doses. In the kidney, parathyroid hormone acts to decrease the renal tubular reabsorption of phosphate and to increase renal tubular

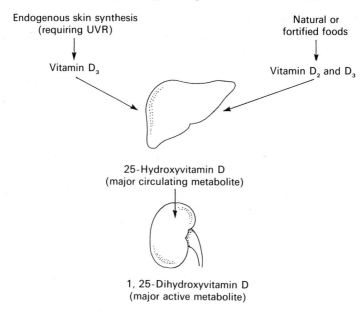

Fig. 1.8. Vitamin D metabolism.

calcium reabsorption. It does not have any direct effect on intestinal calcium absorption, but stimulates it indirectly via activation of renal 1 alpha-hydroxylase, the enzyme which converts 25-hydroxyvitamin D to 1,25-dihydroxyvitamin D.

Vitamin D

Although classically regarded as a vitamin, vitamin D is more accurately described as a steroid hormone which is synthesised in the skin, dietary intake only becoming important when exposure of the skin to ultraviolet irradiation is absent, for example, in the institutionalised and the housebound elderly. On exposure to ultraviolet irradiation, 7-dehydro-cholesterol in the skin is converted to cholecalciferol, or vitamin D_3, which is then transported on a binding protein to the liver, where it undergoes 25-hydroxylation to form the major circulating form of the vitamin, 25-hydroxyvitamin D (Fig. 1.8). Dietary vitamin D may be in the form of cholecalciferol or ergosterol (vitamin D_2); vitamin D_3 occurs naturally in a variety of foods, predominantly oily fish whilst both forms of the vitamin (D_2 and D_3) are used to fortify foods, particularly dairy products.

25-hydroxyvitamin D does not have biological activity at the concentrations normally circulating in plasma but provides a reasonable measure of vitamin D status, providing that the marked seasonal variation in its circulating concentration is taken into account. The major active metabolite, 1,25-dihydroxyvitamin D, is formed by 1 alpha-hydroxylation of 25-hydroxyvitamin D, a reaction which occurs almost solely in the kidney. Circulating levels of the active metabolite are determined by the vitamin D and parathyroid hormone status; in conditions of vitamin D deficiency and increased secretion of parathyroid hormone, the production of 1,25-dihydroxyvitamin D is stimulated, whereas in vitamin D replete states circulating 1,25-dihydroxyvitamin D inhibits its own synthesis.

1,25-dihydroxyvitamin D has diverse biological actions including effects on the cellular proliferation and differentiation of haematopoietic cells, and on mineral metabolism. It stimulates intestinal absorption and renal tubular reabsorption of calcium, and has complex effects on bone. Its ability to promote bone mineralisation in rickets, and osteomalacia is believed to result from the increase in circulating calcium and phosphate levels achieved through increased intestinal absorption and mobilisation from mineralised bone. 1,25-dihydroxyvitamin D also stimulates the production of insulin-like growth factors and osteocalcin and may, under some circumstances, have anabolic effects on bone.

Calcitonin

Calcitonin is a 32 amino-acid peptide, the main source of which are the C cells of the thyroid gland. It is an important inhibitor of osteoclastic bone resorption, a property that is utilised in the treatment of Paget's disease, osteoporosis and hypercalcaemia of malignancy. Its physiological role in humans is uncertain.

Investigation of metabolic bone disease

Clinical history and examination

Careful evaluation of the clinical history and a thorough physical examination are of great value in the diagnosis of metabolic bone disease. Bone pain is a common symptom which may be variable and non-specific, as commonly occurs in osteomalacia, or characteristic, as in some cases of vertebral fracture. Metabolic bone disease is frequently a manifestation of other disorders which can affect one or several systems, and evidence for a past or present history of hepatic, gastrointestinal, renal or endocrine disease should be carefully sought. All drug therapy should be carefully noted since a number of drugs affect calcium and bone homeostasis; these include vitamin D and calcium, thiazides, anticonvulsants, corticosteroids, sex hormones and bile acid binding agents such as cholestyramine. Life-style variables such as cigarette smoking and alcohol should be assessed, and some evaluation of dietary calcium intake should be made, although this can only be approximate. In women, a detailed menstrual history should be taken and details of pregnancies and lactation obtained. The family history is important since some forms of metabolic bone disease are inherited.

Physical examination, together with the history, may reveal the diagnosis in a number of metabolic bone diseases. Rickets can often be recognised by the characteristic skeletal deformities which occur, and in advanced cases of osteomalacia the classical waddling gait and proximal myopathy may reveal the diagnosis. Advanced osteoporosis leads to kyphosis of the dorsal spine and secondary changes in the shape of the abdomen and thorax. Paget's disease can also be diagnosed clinically in advanced cases. Evidence of endocrine or malignant disease should be sought routinely in patients with osteoporosis and signs of renal, hepatic or intestinal disease looked for in those with osteoporosis or osteomalacia. Finally, many of the rarer forms of metabolic bone disease are associated with phenotypic abnormalities which may be diagnostic; these include café-au lait spots (fibrous dysplasia) and blue sclerae (osteogenesis imperfecta).

Although, in some cases, the clinical history and physical examination enable the diagnosis of a metabolic bone disease, further investigation is usually required in order to establish the pathogenesis of the bone disease, and to select the appropriate treatment.

Biochemical investigations

Serum calcium and phosphate

Serum calcium consists of a protein-bound fraction (approximately 40%), an ionised fraction (approximately 48%) and a smaller complexed component (Fig. 1.9). Albumin is the major binding protein for calcium, although small amounts are bound to globulin. In most circumstances the total serum calcium is measured and, when serum albumin and acid/base balance are normal, this provides an adequate assessment of physiologically active (i.e. ionised) calcium. However, if the serum albumin is

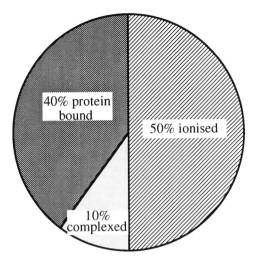

Fig. 1.9. Composition of total serum calcium.

decreased as, for example, in hepatic disease, malabsorption or renal disease, the total serum calcium concentration may be misleading and a correction procedure is necessary to compensate for the changes in serum albumin. A number of correction algorithms have been described and none is consistently accurate; however, a simple rule of thumb is that, for every decrease in serum albumin of 1 g/dl, the total serum calcium should be increased by 0.02 mmol/l. Acidosis is associated with a decrease in the proportion of calcium which is protein bound and hence an increase in the ionised fraction whilst alkalosis has the opposite effects. Other factors which may influence the serum calcium concentration include venostasis, which increases the total concentration because of haemoconcentration and, finally, there is a Circadian rhythm with a maximum amplitude of around 0.125 mmol/l.

Serum phosphorus exists predominantly in an organic form (around 66%) with a smaller inorganic fraction. The circulating phosphate level is affected substantially by dietary intake and by the time of day; the Circadian changes can produce differences of up to 30% in the value obtained. Serum phosphate is also affected by acid/base balance, changes in glucose/insulin status and age. The effects of age are considerable; values in infants are nearly twice as high as in adults, levels falling during childhood to reach adult values by late adolescence.

Blood for serum calcium and phosphate estimation should be obtained without undue stasis and separated promptly, since prolonged standing or haemolysis of the specimen produces an increase in the serum phosphate concentration. Measurement of the serum ionised calcium concentration is seldom necessary in routine clinical practice but is of particular value in seriously ill patients with disturbances of acid/base balance and hypoproteinaemia.

Vitamin D metabolites

Measurement of vitamin D metabolites is of value in certain clinical situations. Serum 25-hydroxyvitamin D concentrations provide an indication of vitamin D status at the time of measurement but must be interpreted in the light of the marked seasonal variation in circulating levels of this metabolite which may result in several-fold differences between winter and summer. Assessment of serum 25-hydroxyvitamin D levels is thus of some value in detecting subjects in high-risk groups, for example, malabsorption, gastrectomy and chronic liver disease, who might benefit from vitamin D prophylaxis but should not be used as a surrogate measure for osteomalacia; mineralisation defects may occur in the presence of normal serum 25-hydroxyvitamin D levels and, conversely, low serum levels may be associated with normal bone histology. Assessment of 25-hydroxyvitamin D levels is also valuable in the diagnosis of iatrogenic or self-imposed vitamin D toxicity (provided that vitamin D itself rather than an active metabolite has been administered). Measurement of 25-hydroxyvitamin and 1,25-dihydroxyvitamin D is useful in the diagnosis of hypocalcaemia associated with abnormal vitamin D metabolism or altered end-organ responsiveness (vitamin D-dependent rickets Type 1 and 11). Finally, in patients with hypercalcaemia and/or hypercalciuria in whom parathyroid hormone secretion is suppressed, high circulating 1,25-dihydroxyvitamin D levels indicate exogenous intoxication with the metabolite or one of its analogues, idiopathic hypercalciuria, or extra-renal production of 1,25-dihydroxyvitamin D associated with granulomatous disease and lymphoma.

Parathyroid hormone

A number of assays for serum parathyroid hormone are available; some of these measure fragments of the molecule (mid-region, N-terminal and C-terminal) whilst others measure the intact hormone. Both the mid-region and intact hormone assay produce elevated serum parathyroid hormone levels in approximately 95% of cases of primary hyperparathyroidism whilst, in non-parathyroid hypercalcaemia, intact parathyroid hormone assays show suppressed values in nearly all cases, although mid-region

Table. 1.3. *Biochemical markers of bone turnover*

Formation	Resorption
Serum: alkaline phosphatase osteocalcin procollagen type 1 peptide	Serum: tartrate-resistant acid phosphatase Urine: calcium hydroxyproline collagen cross-links (pyridinoline + deoxypyridinoline)

assays are less specific. When hypocalcaemia is due to hypoparathyroidism, serum parathyroid hormone levels are undetectable but raised
levels occur in pseudohypoparathyroidism and in secondary hyperparathyroidism. Measurement of serum parathyroid hormone is particularly useful in the evaluation of renal osteodystrophy and its treatment,
levels of the intact hormone only being mildly affected by renal failure.
Secretion of intact parathyroid hormone in normal subjects shows marked
diurnal variation, the highest levels occurring between 0200 and 0600
hours; concentrations outside the reference range may be seen in normal
subjects if blood is collected during this time.

Parathyroid hormone-related peptide

Parathyroid hormone-related peptide is an amino-acid peptide which
shows marked structural homology with parathyroid hormone. It plays an
important role in the pathogenesis of humoral hypercalcaemia of malignancy, being produced by some solid tumours and acting systemically on
bone to increase resorption, thus resulting in hypercalcaemia. Raised
circulating levels of the peptide can be demonstrated in such cases, whereas
undetectable concentrations are found in nearly all cases of primary
hyperparathyroidism.

Biochemical markers of bone turnover

Indirect information about bone formation and resorption can be obtained
from the measurement, in serum or urine, of bone-derived products (Table
1.3). These include serum osteocalcin, alkaline phosphatase and procol-
lagen peptides, which are produced by osteoblasts and are markers of bone
formation and tartrate-resistant acid phosphatase, which is produced
(although not exclusively) by osteoclasts and reflects bone resorption. In

addition, measurement of the urinary excretion of calcium and of collagen breakdown products serve as markers of bone resorption.

Alkaline phosphatase

Serum alkaline phosphatase is the most commonly assessed marker of bone turnover. Total serum alkaline phosphatase reflects the activity of a number of isoenzymes including bone, liver and, during pregnancy, placental; these isoenzymes can be determined separately although this facility is not routinely available. Elevation of serum alkaline phosphatase due to liver disease is associated with raised serum levels of gamma glutamyl transferase and 5-nucleotidase, whereas the activity of these enzymes is normal if elevation of total serum alkaline phosphatase is due solely to the bone isoenzyme.

Alkaline phosphatase activity varies with age, increasing from birth and reaching a maximum during adolescence; thereafter it falls steeply to reach stable values around the end of the second decade. These changes are largely due to changes in production of the bone isoenzyme. Increased serum alkaline phosphatase levels occur during pregnancy, due mainly to an increase in placental isoenzyme. Bone-derived alkaline phosphatase is elevated in a number of metabolic bone diseases, including rickets and osteomalacia, high-turnover osteoporosis, Paget's disease and hyperparathyroid bone disease. Increased levels are also found in many cases of metastatic bone disease. Very low serum alkaline phosphatase levels are found in hypophosphatasia.

Osteocalcin

Osteocalcin is a non-collagenous protein which contains three residues of the vitamin K-dependent amino acid gamma-carboxyglutamic acid and is produced exclusively by osteoblasts. Serum osteocalcin concentrations show qualitatively similar changes during childhood and adolescence as serum alkaline phosphatase but differential changes in the serum concentrations of the two markers sometimes occur in metabolic bone disease, and serum osteocalcin concentrations correlate more closely than alkaline phosphatase activity with bone formation rates. Serum osteocalcin levels are increased in high turnover bone disease and in renal failure, primarily because of decreased clearance. Reduced levels are found in hypoparathyroidism and in conditions associated with low bone turnover, for example, hepatic osteoporosis and rheumatoid arthritis. Assays for the measurement of serum osteocalcin concentrations are not at present widely available for clinical use.

Urinary hydroxyproline and collagen cross-links

Hydroxyproline is derived from collagen breakdown and reflects bone resorption but, since it is not bone specific, urinary excretion may be influenced by extra-skeletal collagen degradation including that ingested in the diet. More recently, the measurement in urine of two collagen cross-linking amino acids, pyridinoline and deoxypyridinoline, has been shown to provide more specific markers of bone resorption. These amino acids form covalent cross-links between adjacent collagen chains in the extracellular matrix; deoxypyridinoline is virtually specific to bone whereas pyridinoline is also found in other connective tissues, notably cartilage. Urinary excretion of deoxypyridinoline and pyridinoline show a Circadian rhythm, the highest levels occurring early in the morning and, unlike hydroxyproline, it is unaffected by dietary intake, thus avoiding the necessity for a gelatin-free diet prior to urinary collection. Urinary excretion of hydroxyproline and collagen cross-links is expressed as a ratio to the urinary concentration of creatinine to correct for possible collection errors.

Increased urinary excretion of hydroxyproline and collagen cross-links is associated with high turnover bone disease, including Paget's disease, hyperparathyroidism and some cases of osteoporosis. Assays for the measurement of urinary hydroxyproline are fairly widely available, but facilities for measuring collagen cross-links are limited to only a small number of centres.

Urinary calcium excretion

Measurement of urinary calcium excretion is valuable in the assessment of some disorders of bone and mineral homeostasis. In normal adults, it is usually in the range of 2.5–6.25 mmol/24 hours (100–250 mg) but lower values are obtained in vitamin D deficiency and osteomalacia, chronic renal disease, familial hypercalciuric hypercalcaemia, hypoparathyroidism and thiazide ingestion. Hypercalciuria occurs in conditions associated with high turnover bone disease and in sarcoidosis, primary hyper-parathyroidism, renal tubular acidosis, metastatic bone disease and idiopathic hypercalciuria.

Bone densitometry

The diagnosis and management of osteoporosis has been greatly advanced by the development of non-invasive techniques which assess bone density

Table. 1.4. *Measurement of bone mass*

Method	Site	Precision
Single photon absorptiometry	Radius	1–2%
Dual photon absorptiometry	Spine, femur, whole body	2–3%
Dual energy X-ray absorptiometry	Spine, femur, whole body, os calcis, radius	0.5–3.0%
Broadband ultrasonic attenuation	Os calcis, patella	3–5%

at sites of clinical relevance such as the radius, hip and spine (Table 1.4). These techniques include single and dual photon absorptiometry, quantitative computed tomography, broadband ultrasonic attenuation and dual energy X-ray absorptiometry; because of its extremely low radiation dose and ability rapidly to assess axial bone mass, dual energy X-ray absorptiometry is the method of choice. With the exception of quantitative computed tomography, the techniques listed do not measure true bone density but relate bone mineral content to a given area. The resulting value is expressed in grams/cm² and reflects an areal rather than a volume density. Since the third dimension of size, depth, is ignored in the calculation of areal density, the values obtained are to some extent dependent on bone size and hence body size.

The term osteopenia is generally used to describe low bone mineral density, whether assessed densitometrically or radiologically, and is not synonymous with osteoporosis. In particular, osteomalacia may be associated with reduced bone mineral density because of the increase in amount of unmineralised bone which characterises this condition. It is therefore important to exclude osteomalacia when osteopenia is demonstrated in high risk groups, for example, in patients with malabsorption, chronic renal failure and privational vitamin D deficiency.

Single and dual photon absorptiometry

Single photon absorptiometry has been available for many years and is limited to measurements of appendicular bone mass, usually in the radius. Measurements at this site reflect both cortical and trabecular bone mass, values obtained for the distal forearm predominantly reflecting trabecular bone mass and those at more proximal sites cortical bone mass. The technique is based on transmission measurements through tissues of a monoenergetic energy source, usually [125]iodine, differential photon absorption between bone and soft tissue enabling calculation of bone mineral content, usually expressed as a ratio to bone width in grams/cm².

The use of a dual energy photon source enables simultaneous transmission measurements through bone and soft tissue; the technique can thus be applied to the axial skeleton, but has now been superseded by dual energy X-ray absorptiometry.

Quantitative computed tomography

Quantitative computed tomography is based on the comparison of CT values in bone with those of a compound with an attenuation coefficient similar to that of bone mineral. It has been most widely applied to the spine although it can also be used for measurements in the appendicular skeleton. It possesses the ability to measure trabecular bone density only but its use is limited by its expense and by the radiation dose involved.

Broadband ultrasonic attenuation

Broadband ultrasonic attenuation has been applied to the os calcis and the patella, both sites of predominantly trabecular bone; both bone mass and architecture influence the value obtained although their relative contributions have not been accurately assessed. Values for broadband ultrasonic attenuation in the os calcis show a similar discrimination between osteoporotic and normal subjects as bone density measurements elsewhere in the skeleton and may also have similar predictive value for fracture risk, although this is disputed. The technique is relatively cheap and is radiation free.

Dual energy X-ray absorptiometry

Over the past few years, dual energy X-ray absorptiometry (DXA) has become the method of choice for measurements of bone mass in the spine and the femur (Figs. 1.10, 1.11). The radiation dose required is less than the average natural daily background radiation, and measurements can be made rapidly. Measurements are made in the lumbar spine, usually in the second, third and fourth lumbar vertebrae. Osteophyte formation, extra-skeletal calcification, and vertebral deformity, may all lead to falsely elevated values for bone density; furthermore, it should be noted that normal vertebral morphology and bone density in the lumbar spine do not necessarily exclude osteoporotic changes in the dorsal spine, since differential changes may occur in a number of conditions including post-menopausal osteoporosis and corticosteroid-induced osteoporosis. The precision of the technique is slightly superior to or comparable with that of other methods, in vivo precision of 1–2% being quoted for the spine, and 1.5–3.0% for the femur, although it is worse for measurements of low bone density.

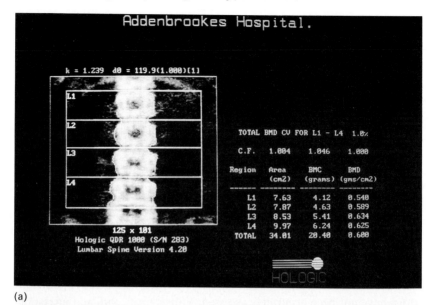

(a)

(b)

Fig. 1.10. Dual energy X-ray absorptiometry of the spine: (*a*) image obtained of lumbar spine, (*b*) the value obtained is displayed in relation to the age- and sex-matched reference range.

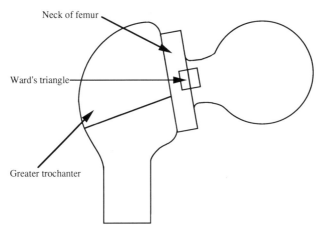

Fig. 1.11. Dual energy X-ray absorptiometry: the three areas of measurement in the femur.

Radiological evaluation of bone disease

Radiology of the skeleton is widely used in the assessment of metabolic bone disease, particularly in the diagnosis of Paget's disease and metastatic bone disease. Although of limited value in the diagnosis of osteoporosis, it is of considerable value in assessing the degree of vertebral deformity present and in determining changes during the course of treatment. Radiological abnormalities associated with osteomalacia are very variable and, in general, pathognomonic changes occur only in advanced disease, although even then they are not invariable. In contrast, radiological changes appear relatively early in the course of rickets and are more characteristic, although other conditions such as copper deficiency, hypophosphatasia and fluorosis can mimic these changes. Renal osteodystrophy may result in a number of radiological abnormalities including osteopenia, osteosclerosis, fractures and subperiosteal erosion. Finally, radiological evaluation forms the main diagnostic technique for a number of rare genetic and acquired forms of bone disease.

Assessment of bone mass from radiographs is notoriously inaccurate, and bone loss of around 50% is required before it can be reliably detected by this approach. Semi-quantitative techniques have been developed to assess cortical and medullary width in the metacarpals; these were widely used for the assessment of osteoporosis before the advent of more sophisticated techniques. Changes in the trabecular pattern can be detected in some forms of metabolic bone disease, but are not always reliable or specific.

Isotope bone scanning

Technetium-labelled bisphosphonate compounds are widely used in the clinical evaluation of a number of conditions including metastatic bone disease and primary bone tumours, Paget's disease, osteomalacia and hyperparathyroid bone disease. Technetium 99m is a gamma emitter with a gamma ray energy which makes it well suited for gamma camera imaging. The isotope is administered intravenously and gamma camera imaging is performed approximately 2–3 hours after injection; 24-hour whole body retention of the isotope can also be assessed. Isotope bone scanning is of most value in the diagnosis of primary and secondary bone tumours; in metabolic bone disease, the commonest abnormality is increased skeletal uptake of the isotope, a non-specific indication of increased bone turnover. The technique has no role to play in the diagnosis of osteoporosis, but may be valuable in the diagnosis of focal abnormalities associated with the condition, such as micro-fractures and fluoride-associated stress fractures, in which radiology may be negative.

Histological investigations

When clinical, biochemical, and radiological evidence of bone disease is absent or conflicting, examination of bone histology may be required for the diagnosis of metabolic bone disease. In particular, it may be indicated to confirm or exclude a diagnosis of osteomalacia or to differentiate between the several forms of renal osteodystrophy. The preparation of undecalcified bone histological sections and their interpretation are not routinely available, although there are a number of centres in the UK with such facilities where cases can be referred.

Iliac crest bone biopsy

Bone biopsy is a safe procedure which is normally performed on an out-patient basis under mild sedation and local anaesthesia. The patient is placed supine on a bed or couch and a short acting sedative, such as midazolam, 2.5–5.0 mg, is injected intravenously. The approach most commonly used is trans-iliac, a core 6–8 mm in diameter being obtained approximately one inch below and behind the anterior superior iliac spine; the biopsy contains cortical bone at both ends and trabecular bone between. Using a thin trocar and stilette, the periosteum over both the outer and inner cortex is anaesthesised using 1% lignocaine; if this is

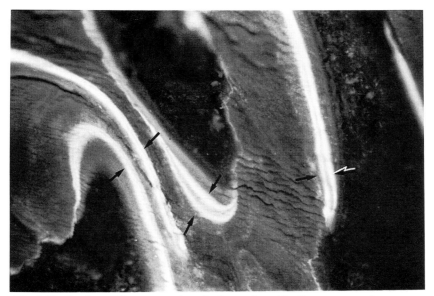

Fig. 1.12. Section of iliac crest trabecular bone viewed by fluorescence microscopy to show double tetracycline labels (arrowed).

adequately performed, the procedure is not painful, although some soreness after the biopsy is common and usually lasts for about 24 hours. The complication rate of bone biopsy is very low; in one large series, it was less than 0.5%, the commonest problem being haematoma. There is no reported mortality from the procedure.

After the biopsy has been taken, it is placed in preservative (buffered formalin or 70% alcohol), processed and subsequently embedded in a hard medium such as methylmethacrylate. Undecalcified sections are cut using a special microtome and stained to demonstrate mineralised bone, un-mineralised bone (osteoid), and bone cells. At the interface between mineralised and unmineralised bone, calcification fronts can be demonstrated, either using stains such as toluidine blue or by tetracycline fluorescence in unstained sections following administration of tetracycline prior to the biopsy (Fig. 1.12). The technique of double tetracycline labelling, in which two, time-spaced doses are given before the biopsy, is widely used in research to enable measurement or calculation of dynamic indices related to bone formation, but is not routinely required for clinical purposes. However, a single tetracycline label should be given 48 hours before the biopsy whenever possible to identify calcification fronts, since toluidine blue staining may not always be reliable in this respect. The most widely used preparation is demethylchlortetracycline, usually given in two doses of 300 mg.

Bone biopsy is widely used as a research procedure to characterise cellular and structural abnormalities associated with bone disease, and to assess the mechanisms by which drugs affect bone. In these circumstances, double tetracyline labelling should always be used to maximise the information obtained. The usual labelling regime is 2 days of label, 10 days free, 2 days of label; the biopsy is performed 5 days after the second day of the last label. A suitable regimen for the four label days is demethylchlortetracycline, 300 mg twice daily.

Histological features of metabolic bone disease

Osteomalacia

The cardinal feature of osteomalacia is defective mineralisation, resulting in increased amounts of osteoid or unmineralised bone, and reduced or absent calcification fronts. The mineralisation defect leads to an increase in the width of osteoid seams and in the amount of osteoid relative to mineralised bone; this must be distinguished from the increase in surface extent of osteoid which is associated with increased bone turnover, from whatever cause. Strict histological diagnostic criteria for osteomalacia are an increase in osteoid seam width greater than 2 standard deviations above the normal mean value, and an increase in mineralisation lag time, calculated from the mean wall width, which represents the average amount of bone formed per remodelling unit, divided by the bone formation rate at cellular level. In clinical practice, quantitative assessment is rarely, if ever, necessary and the diagnosis of osteomalacia can usually be made on the basis of qualitative assessment of osteoid seam width and calcification fronts. A mean osteoid seam width of 15 µm or more is regarded as abnormally high, whilst calcification fronts associated with less than 50–60% of the osteoid covered surface would be abnormally low. Occasionally, focal osteomalacia may be present; this is seen in some patients treated for Paget's disease with the bisphosphonate etidronate and is characterised by the presence of occasional thick osteoid seams which are mostly unassociated with calcification fronts, although osteoid seams of normal width, and with normal calcification fronts, are also seen.

Osteoporosis

Iliac crest bone biopsy is an insensitive diagnostic technique for osteoporosis because of the skeletal heterogeneity of this disease and the failure of iliac crest bone reliably to reflect changes in more clinically relevant skeletal sites such as the spine and femur; bone volume in the iliac crest may be normal in the presence of severe spinal osteoporosis with multiple fractures. However, because osteomalacia may be associated with radiological and densitometric abnormalities indistinguishable from those of osteoporosis, bone biopsy may be indicated to exclude osteomalacia in high risk cases, for example, in patients with malabsorption, gastrectomy or suspected or proven privational vitamin D deficiency.

Renal osteodystrophy

Renal osteodystrophy is a complex disorder in which varying combinations of osteomalacia, secondary hyperparathyroidism, osteosclerosis and osteoporosis may occur. Bone biopsy is often necessary to evaluate the relative contributions of these abnormalities in order to determine the most appropriate therapy. Secondary hyperparathyroidism is the most common form of bone disease and leads to an increase in bone turnover and increased depth of resorption cavities, 'tunnelling resorption' often being encountered in the middle of trabecular plates. The number of osteoclasts and osteoblasts is increased, and the high rate of bone turnover leads to the formation of woven bone and paratrabecular fibrosis (osteitis fibrosa). Osteomalacia associated with renal dysfunction may be due to vitamin D deficiency, aluminium excess or hypophosphataemia; it is characterised histologically by an increase in osteoid seam width, and by decreased mineralisation leading to absent or greatly reduced calcification fronts and tetracycline uptake. Bone turnover is reduced and, in cases where aluminium excess is responsible, it can be demonstrated histologically in bone sections at the osteoid/mineralised bone interface. Finally, some symptomatic patients develop 'aplastic' bone disease in which osteoid amount is normal and bone turnover is greatly reduced. The pathogenesis of this form of bone disease is not clearly understood, although in some cases it may be related to aluminium toxicity.

Further reading

Anderson, D.C. (1990). Hormones and the skeleton. In *Osteoporosis*. ed. R. Smith. Royal College of Physicians of London, Oxprint Ltd, Oxford, England, pp. 79–90.

Lang, P., Stieger, P., Faulkner, K., Gluer, C. & Genant, H.K. (1991). Osteoporosis: current techniques and recent developments in quantitive bone densitometry. *Radiology Clinics of North America* **29**, 49–76.

Parfitt, A.M. (1984). The cellular basis of bone remodelling. The quantum concept re-examined in the light of recent advances in cell biology of bone. *Calcified Tissue Internat.* **36**, S37–45.

Recker, R., ed. (1983). *Bone Histomorphometry. Techniques and Interpretations.* CRC Press Inc, Boca Raton.

Russell, R.G.G. (1990). Bone cell biology: the role of cytokines and other mediators. In *Osteoporosis.* ed. R. Smith. Royal College of Physicians of London, Oxprint Ltd, Oxford, England, pp. 9–43.

2

Osteoporosis

Definition, prevalence and epidemiology

Definition

Osteoporosis is characterised by reduced bone mass and by increased risk of fragility fracture. The term osteopenia is used to describe a reduction in bone mass whilst osteoporosis generally denotes the presence of fracture. Fragility fractures are defined as fractures occurring after a fall from standing height or less and may occur without any obvious preceding trauma. The three most common fracture sites in osteoporosis are the spine, the femoral neck and the radius, but fractures may also occur at a number of other sites, particularly the pelvis and humerus.

Prevalence and epidemiology

Fragility fractures constitute an enormous public health problem in the Western world, and are a major cause of morbidity and mortality in the elderly population. In the United Kingdom it is estimated that osteoporosis is responsible for at least 250000 fractures annually, and in the United States the corresponding figure is estimated at 1.3 million. The calculated life-time risk of vertebral fracture in white, post-menopausal women is estimated to be over 30%; for Colles' and hip fracture it is between 10 and 15%. The costs of these fractures to the health services are difficult to quantify accurately but are believed to be at least £500 million in the United Kingdom and $7.3 billion in the USA.

The incidence of fragility fractures increases with age, exponentially for vertebral and hip fractures whilst Colles' fractures plateau around the age of 60. Evidence for an increase in the age-specific incidence of hip fracture over the past few decades has been reported from the United States and

from a number of European countries although these rising rates may now
be stabilising. However, because of the expected increase in the number of
elderly people in the population, the number of osteoporotic fractures can
be expected to rise by 50% over the next 20 years unless major advances are
made in prevention of the disease. The incidence of hip fracture shows large
geographical variation, being low in some Negroid populations and much
higher in American and European whites.

Hip fractures

Hip fractures affect approximately one in three women and one in six men
surviving to extreme old age, the highest incidence being between the ages
of 75 and 85 years. Mortality is high, being around 15–20% at six months,
and the majority of survivors show increased dependency, sometimes
necessitating institutionalisation. Hospital admission is often prolonged
because of the advanced age and frailty of many hip fracture sufferers, and
the consequent high incidence of post-operative complications causes
occupation of a considerable proportion of orthopaedic hospital beds and
high costs. Nearly all hip fractures are preceded by a fall; since low bone
mass is virtually universal in extreme old age, the risk of falling and the
associated protective responses are major determinants of this type of
fracture.

Vertebral fractures

The incidence of vertebral fracture is unknown; since a large proportion,
perhaps as many as 60–70% of such fractures, are asymptomatic or
insufficiently painful to lead to medical consultation, incidence rates
cannot be accurately established from hospital records as with hip and
wrist fractures. Furthermore, vertebral fractures are less easy to define than
hip fractures, and prevalence rates are critically dependent upon the criteria
used. When defined as a reduction in vertebral height of 20% or more, one
study from the UK reported an overall prevalence of 7.8% in women aged
between 50 and 80 years (mean 64.4). The male to female ratio of vertebral
fractures is usually quoted at around seven to one but in truth it is unknown
and some data indicate that vertebral fractures may be more common in
men than formerly believed. The morbidity and financial cost of vertebral
fractures have received little attention but are likely to be considerable.

Wrist fractures

Colles' fractures typically occur after falling forwards onto the outstetched
hand and are most commonly associated with outside falls, particularly
during winter snow and ice. The incidence of these fractures rises rapidly in

Table. 2.1. *Main features of Type I and Type II osteoporosis*

	Type 1	Type 2
Age (year)	50–75	70+
Sex ratio (F:M)	6:1	2:1
Type of bone loss	Mainly trabecular	Trabecular + cortical
Fracture sites	Vertebrae + radius	Vertebrae + hip

the immediate post-menopausal period and reaches a peak at around 55–60 years of age. Although these fractures seldom have devastating long-term consequences, they require hospital treatment and may cause considerable inconvenience to the sufferer, with residual functional disability and discomfort for some months after fracture. Some degree of deformity of the wrist is a common and permanent consequence of these fractures.

Pathogenesis

Osteoporosis is a multifactorial disease although, in women, oestrogen deficiency is usually pivotal. In women, the division of most cases of primary osteoporosis into post-menopausal and senile has been replaced by Type 1 and Type 11 osteoporosis, the former corresponding to post-menopausal osteoporosis and being characterised by mainly trabecular bone loss, leading to fractures of the spine and radius, whereas in Type 11 osteoporosis both cortical and trabecular bone loss occur, resulting in more hip fractures and corresponding to senile osteoporosis (Table 2.1). It is postulated that oestrogen deficiency is the main pathogenetic factor in Type 1 osteoporosis whilst vitamin D deficiency and secondary hyper-parathyroidism play an important role in the development of Type 11 osteoporosis. In reality, both of these mechanisms are likely to operate in many women, and the age at which fracture occurs may be related more to peak bone mass than to specific pathogenetic factors.

A number of endogenous and exogenous factors affect bone mass; these include genetically determined characteristics, life-style variables, diseases and drugs. Genetic influences probably operate through effects on peak bone mass, whilst the remaining life-style, disease and pharmacological factors may affect both peak bone mass and/or age-related bone loss.

Endogenous risk factors (Table 2.2)

The most important endogenous risk factors for osteoporosis are advanced age, female sex and Caucasian or Asian race. Genetic factors are also

Table. 2.2. *Endogenous risk factors for osteoporosis*	Table. 2.3. *Major exogenous risk factors for osteoporosis*
Female sex	Premature menopause
Advanced age	Pre-menopausal amenorrhoea
Caucasian/Asian race	Hypercortisolism
Small body build	Hyperthyroidism
	Bowel disease/malabsorption

important in so far as they determine body build and bone size, although a family history of osteoporosis is a relatively weak risk factor. Obesity appears to be protective.

Exogenous risk factors (Table 2.3)

A number of exogenous risk factors have been defined; of these the most important are premature menopause or pre-menopausal oophorectomy, other causes of pre-menopausal oestrogen deficiency such as anorexia nervosa, excessive physical exercise and chronic illness, malabsorption and, finally, long-term corticosteroid therapy. In addition, overtreatment of hypothyroidism with thyroxine may be a risk factor for osteoporosis. Conversely, thiazide administration appears to have protective effects on femoral bone mass and hip fracture risk. The causes of secondary osteoporosis are shown in Table 2.4; in men, secondary causes may account for as many as 55% of all cases of osteoporosis whereas in women, only 10–20% can be attributed to such causes.

Risk factors for falling are particularly important determinants of hip fracture and include impaired cognitive, neuromuscular and visual function and the use of sedative medications and alcohol. Environmental risk factors for falling, such as loose carpeting, uneven pavements and steps, slippery floor surfaces, etc also contribute.

Life-style risk factors (Table 2.4)

Life-style variables which may affect bone mass include alcohol ingestion, cigarette smoking, physical activity and dietary habits, particularly calcium intake. Excessive alcohol ingestion is associated with reduced bone mass and increased fracture risk; in addition to possible direct adverse effects of alcohol on bone, factors such as malnutrition, liver disease and increased propensity to fall contribute to osteoporosis in such subjects. Whether moderate alcohol consumption also has adverse effects on bone mass is less certain. The effects of tobacco may also be mediated by a combination of

Table. 2.4. *Life-style variables
affecting bone mass*

Alcohol
Cigarettes
Physical activity
Calcium intake
Vitamin D status

direct and indirect effects, the latter including decreased body weight, concurrent alcohol consumption and, in women, earlier age at menopause. Physical activity may influence peak bone mass and age-related bone loss although any benefit is likely to be related to those parts of the skeleton subjected to weight-bearing stresses and excessive exercise in women can lead to amenorrhoea and bone loss, as occurs in elite female athletes and ballet dancers. Finally, nutritional factors affect bone mass; body weight is a major determinant of bone mass, low weight being a risk factor for osteoporosis and obesity being protective. The influence of dietary calcium intake is more controversial although there is some evidence that it is positively related to peak bone mass, and a number of studies have shown that calcium supplementation reduces age-related bone loss; a convincing association between calcium intake and fracture risk, however, has not been demonstrated. Vitamin D deficiency, which is relatively common in the elderly UK population, may lead to secondary hyperparathyroidism, with a consequent increase in cortical bone loss.

Diagnosis of osteoporosis

The clinical manifestations of osteoporosis appear late in the course of the disease after years, often decades, of bone loss; treatment of the established condition is therefore unsatisfactory and significant impact on morbidity and mortality can only be achieved through prevention, requiring early diagnosis at a stage when bone loss is minimal. The ultimate aim of any preventive strategy is to reduce fracture risk and, if universal treatment is to be avoided, diagnostic techniques should be aimed at selecting those subjects at greatest risk from fracture.

Clinical manifestations

Clinical symptoms and signs in osteoporosis are related to fracture, although the occurrence of back pain in some patients with low bone mass and no radiologically demonstrable fracture raises the question of whether

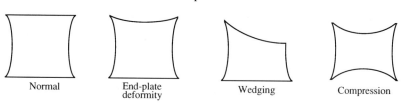

Fig. 2.1. Types of vertebral deformity associated with osteoporosis. (Reproduced by permission of the Oxford University Press.)

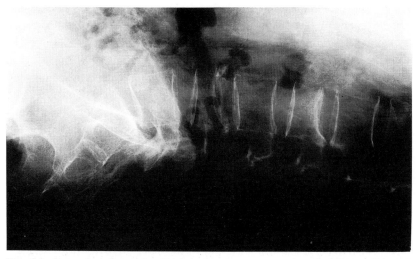

Fig. 2.2. Lateral radiograph of spine showing compression fracture at L4 and deformity at L2.

microfractures (fractures of individual bone trabeculae) may also give rise to pain. In view of the high prevalence of back pain in the population, and the multitude of possible causal factors, causes other than osteoporosis should always be sought and, when possible, excluded.

The term vertebral fracture is generally used to describe either a wedge or a crush deformity (Fig. 2.1). The precise definition of vertebral fracture is the subject of some controversy but a reasonable working rule is a reduction in anterior, middle or posterior height of 25% or more, a change which can normally be detected on qualitative assessment of a radiograph (Fig. 2.2). The symptoms attributable to these two fracture types have not been clearly defined although crush fractures probably cause severe, acute pain more frequently than wedge fractures. Vertebral fractures occur most commonly at the dorsolumbar junction (D12 and L1) and in the mid-dorsal spine, compression fractures being most common at the former location and wedge deformity at the latter.

Vertebral fractures may be asymptomatic but in at least one-third of cases cause sudden, severe back pain at the level of the fracture, the pain often radiating anteriorly around the thorax or abdomen. This pain generally improves over the ensuing months or even years; however, the natural history of pain after vertebral fracture is extremely variable, some patients being pain-free after a few months whilst, in others, pain persists indefinitely. Spinal cord compression is virtually never associated with osteoporotic vertebral fractures, and the presence of neurological symptoms and/or signs should alert the clinician to other diagnoses such as Paget's disease or bone metastases. Multiple fractures lead to height loss, spinal deformity, protruberance of the abdomen and, in extreme cases, pain due to friction between the lower ribs and the iliac crest.

The morbidity of vertebral fractures has not been established but is likely to be considerable. Pain, height loss and spinal deformity may result in severe disability and restriction of many normal activities. Loss of confidence often occurs after falls and/or fractures, leading to an even greater reduction in activity, and the alterations in body shape associated with spinal osteoporosis cause inconvenience and distress.

Biochemistry

Conventional biochemical tests are usually normal in osteoporosis, although plasma alkaline phosphatase levels may be elevated immediately after fracture has occurred. Measurement of markers of bone turnover provide information about whole body rates of remodelling, but at present these tests are not routinely available. Biochemical investigation is particularly important in the exclusion of secondary causes of osteoporosis (see below).

Radiology

Radiology plays an important role in the diagnosis and evaluation of established osteoporosis. Lateral X-rays of the lumbar and dorsal spine provide the only reliable means of detecting vertebral deformities and also provide a baseline on which to judge the effects of treatment on fracture rate. Radiological evaluation of bone mass is highly subjective and therefore unreliable; however, unequivocal radiological osteopenia is a sign of advanced bone mineral loss.

Bone densitometry

The development of safe, non-invasive and precise techniques for the measurement of bone mineral density at sites of clinical relevance such as

Table. 2.5. *Causes of secondary osteoporosis*

Endocrine	hypercortisolism
	hyperthyroidism
	hyperprolactinaemia
	hypergonadism
	hyperparathyroidism
Neoplasia/marrow disorders	myeloma
	leukaemia
	lymphoma
	mastocytosis
	lipoidoses
Drug-related	corticosteroids
	heparin
	anticonvulsants
	thyroxine
	alcohol
Connective tissue disorders	osteogenesis imperfecta
	Ehlers–Danlos syndrome
	Marfan's syndrome
	homocystinuria
	Menke's syndrome
Others	immobilisation
	bowel disease/malabsorption
	chronic liver disease
	gastric surgery
	chronic renal disease
	post-transplantation

the spine, hip and radius has led to considerable improvement in the diagnosis and clinical management of osteoporosis. These techniques, which are described in the first chapter, have both proven and potential applications; in the former category are their use in clinical practice whilst their value in screening susceptible subgroups of the population to define future fracture risk remains unproven and controversial. These applications are considered in detail in the next section.

Differential diagnosis of osteoporosis

An essential part of investigation of the osteoporotic patient is the exclusion of secondary causes (Table 2.5). A blood count, erythrocyte sedimentation rate (ESR), urea and electrolytes and liver function tests should be performed routinely, together with protein immunoelectrophoresis, examination of the urine for Bence-Jones proteins and, finally, thyroid function tests. If clinical or radiological evidence suggests malignant disease, an isotope bone scan should be carried out and since 10% of patients with myeloma may have normal protein immunoelectrophoresis and no Bence-Jones proteinuria, bone marrow biopsy should be performed if there is a high index of clinical suspicion.

In men, the high proportion of cases with secondary causes demands rigorous investigation. In addition to the tests detailed above, serum testosterone and gonadotrophins should be measured and, in the presence of low serum testosterone and low or normal gonadotrophins, serum prolactin should be assessed. Hypogonadism may not always be clinically overt and serum testosterone may be within the normal range, elevated gonadotrophins providing the only evidence. Hypercortisolism should be excluded since it may occasionally present with clinical signs of osteoporosis before other manifestations of corticosteroid excess appear; measurement of urinary cortisol excretion is probably the investigation of choice. Alcohol abuse is a common factor in male osteoporosis and is not always accompanied by clinical or biochemical evidence of liver disease. Urinary calcium excretion should be measured in 24-hour samples and the fasting urinary calcium/creatinine ratio assessed to determine whether there is evidence of idiopathic hypercalciuria. Conditions such as osteogenesis imperfecta, Ehlers–Danlos and Marfan's syndrome can usually be diagnosed on the basis of clinical examination and family history. In patients with a history of malabsorption, chronic liver disease or gastrectomy, it may be necessary to perform a bone biopsy in order to exclude osteomalacia.

Exclusion of secondary causes of osteoporosis is also important in younger women presenting with osteopenia and/or fragility fracture. Since osteopenia is such a common occurrence in elderly women detailed investigation in such cases is unlikely to be cost-effective, but common secondary causes of osteoporosis should be excluded in all women presenting with a fragility fracture.

Assessment of bone mass

Age-related changes in bone mass (Fig. 2.3)

Age-related bone loss affects both men and women and occurs in cortical and trabecular bone throughout the skeleton. The rate and onset of bone loss differs between cortical and trabecular bone and also varies between different skeletal sites. In women, it is estimated that approximately 35% and 50% of cortical and trabecular bone, respectively, are lost over a

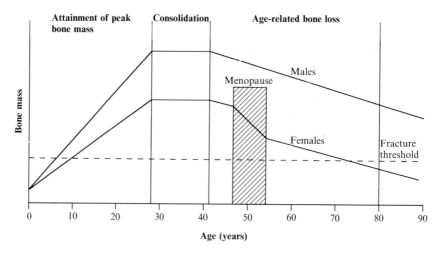

Fig. 2.3. Age-related changes in bone mass: schematic representation. (Reproduced with permission of the Editor of *Clinical Endocrinology*.)

lifetime; in men, bone loss is around two-thirds of this amount. The highest rates of bone loss occur in trabecular bone which has a higher surface to volume ratio and hence a greater capacity for rapid bone loss.

Peak bone mass is thought to be achieved during the third decade of life, following which there may be a period of consolidation before the onset of age-related bone loss. Peak bone mass is a major determinant of bone mass and fracture risk in later life and is influenced by genetic, nutritional, mechanical and hormonal factors. The onset of age-related bone loss has not been accurately established; some studies indicate that pre-menopausal bone loss occurs whilst others have demonstrated bone loss only in peri- or post-menopausal women. In women, increased rates of bone loss during the menopause have been demonstrated, rates in the spine being around 2–3% per annum and between 1 and 2% at the radius and femur. After the age of 60 years or so, bone loss decreases and may eventually cease in later years. Most studies of age-related bone loss have been carried out in women, and the changes in men are not well characterised; however, there does not appear to be an increase in the rate of bone loss equivalent to that occurring during the menopause.

Peak bone mass is closely related to body size and is generally greater in men than in women. This, together with the acceleration in bone loss which occurs during the menopause and the greater longevity of women, contributes to the higher incidence of osteoporosis in women than in men.

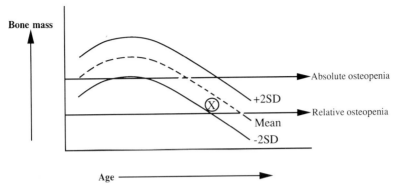

Fig. 2.4. The concepts of absolute and relative osteopenia. The bone mineral density value marked X is within two standard deviations of the mean reference age-matched value but below that of young adults. This represents absolute osteopenia but not relative osteopenia.

Definition of osteopenia

Although the term osteopenia is sometimes associated with reduced radiodensity on X-rays, nowadays it is used more specifically to denote reduced bone mineral density as assessed by dual energy X-ray absorptiometry or other densitometric techniques. The term relative osteopenia is used when bone mass is reduced relative to age-matched normal values whilst absolute osteopenia denotes a reduction in bone mass relative to young normal values (Fig. 2.4). The concept of a fracture threshold is useful in some respects but the threshold value, expressed in absolute terms, varies according to skeletal site, and most elderly women and many elderly men with no fracture have bone mass values below this level; this approach also requires standardisation of all densitometers. Comparison of bone density with age- and sex-matched control values is useful when comparing disease populations at risk from osteoporosis (e.g. thyrotoxicosis, malabsorption) with the normal population but the discrimination of those at risk from fracture is poor in elderly populations because of the considerable overlap in values between fracture and non-fracture cases. The best discrimination between fracture and non-fracture cases is probably provided by comparison of bone density values with sex-matched young normal subjects. However, it is important to recognise that osteoporotic fractures of the dorsal spine may sometimes occur in association with normal lumbar spine radiology and densitometry; in patients at high risk from osteoporosis or in whom clinical signs of dorsal spine involvement are present, lateral X-rays of the dorsal spine should be performed in addition to bone densitometry.

Standard scores (Z scores) are most commonly used to express bone density values at any given site; these represent the difference between the observed value and the mean value of the reference population divided by the standard deviation of the reference population. For relative osteopenia, the mean and standard deviation of age-matched controls is used whilst young normal mean and standard deviation values are used for absolute osteopenia. The expression of bone density as Z scores overcomes the problems of using absolute bone density values, which are technique- and machine-dependent and automatically takes into account age and sex-related changes in the reference population at any given site.

Bone mass and fracture risk

Bone mass is a major determinant of bone strength and fracture risk, but the considerable overlap in bone density values between fracture and non-fracture cases points to the importance of other factors in the pathogenesis of fracture, particularly since bone mass in fracture cases may be underestimated because of acceleration of bone loss after fracture as a result of reduced physical activity. The most important of these is trauma, which virtually always precedes fractures of the radius and hip and sometimes also contributes to vertebral fracture. Other determinants of bone strength and fracture risk include trabecular bone microstructure, the physico-chemical composition of organic and non-organic components of bone and the rate of bone turnover, which determines bone age and microfracture repair.

A number of prospective studies have demonstrated that a single measurement of bone mass is related to future fracture risk but the strength of this relationship is controversial. All these studies have been carried out in women and have mainly been based on bone mass measurements in the radius, although some have also included measurements in the spine and os calcis. The data from these studies show clearly that decreasing bone mass is associated with an increasing gradient of fracture risk, a decrease of one standard deviation in bone mass increasing the relative risk of fracture to between 1.5 and 2.5; the presence of a pre-existing vertebral fracture substantially and independently further increases future fracture risk. With increasing age, bone mass becomes a less important determinant of fracture risk, probably because in a population in which low bone mass is almost universal, the risk of falling will largely determine fracture risk. There are,

Table. 2.6. *Clinical indications for bone densitometry*

Radiological evidence of osteopenia ± vertebral fracture
Long-term corticosteroid therapy
Pre-menopausal amenorrhoea
Intestinal disease/malabsorption

however, relatively few prospective data relating bone mass at the menopause to future fracture risk; if the rates of bone loss during and immediately after the menopause show large variations between individual women, menopausal bone mass might be less strongly predictive of fracture risk than bone mass measured some years later. Alternatively, the variability in rates of bone loss which have been demonstrated over relatively short time periods may be attributable to the phasic nature of bone loss, the absolute magnitude of bone loss over longer periods being quantitatively similar.

The question of whether fracture risk at a particular site is best predicted by assessment of bone mass at that site is controversial but there is increasing evidence that, at least for hip fracture, femoral neck bone density is more strongly related to future fracture risk than bone density measured at sites such as the spine or radius. Although correlations between bone mass at different skeletal sites are generally statistically significant, they are insufficiently strong to be predictive reflecting, amongst other factors, the heterogeneity of bone loss in osteoporosis. In reality, the site of measurement is dictated by the resources available and any advantage offered by dual energy X-ray absorptiometry has to be weighed against the practical and financial advantages of single photon absorptiometry or broadband ultrasonic attenuation.

Clinical indications for bone mass measurement (Table 2.6)

Bone densitometry has become an important tool in the clinical management of osteoporosis. Measurement of bone mass is useful both in the diagnosis of osteoporosis and in assessing the response to treatment, but it is not always necessary and should only be undertaken if the result obtained will influence patient management. Indications for bone densitometry include radiological evidence of osteopenia and/or vertebral deformity; however, falsely high values occur in those with vertebral deformity affecting the lumbar spine and in elderly subjects with osteophyte formation and extra-skeletal calcification. Long-term corticosteroid therapy in women or men is also an indication for bone densitometry because of the high risk of osteoporosis in such subjects. In women with a menopause before the age of 40 years, hormone replacement therapy should be given routinely, and bone densitometry is not generally required, although the demonstration of low bone mass may be useful in persuading those who are reluctant to take hormone replacement therapy; conversely, women in whom relative contraindications to such therapy exist may be reassured by the finding of normal bone mass, although in high risk cases bone densitometry should be repeated at intervals of one to two years. Other high risk groups in whom bone densitometry should be performed include those with secondary amenorrhoea, women in whom the menopause occurs between 40 and 45 years of age and patients with intestinal disease and malabsorption. The recommendation, by some, that bone densitometry should be performed in all patients with primary hyperparathyroidism cannot be justified on the basis of present evidence; however, the increasing evidence that long-term thyroxine replacement therapy may have adverse effects on bone mass indicates that bone densitometry should be considered in such patients, particularly when other risk factors are present.

Screening for osteoporosis

Bone densitometry

The relationship in retrospective and prospective studies between bone mass and fracture, the ability to measure bone mass by non-invasive techniques and the beneficial effects of hormone replacement therapy on bone mass and fracture risk have raised the possibility of mass screening for all peri-menopausal women, based on bone mass measurements. Such an approach cannot, however, be justified at present for a number of reasons. First, there is insufficient knowledge about the predictive value of bone mass measurement at the menopause for fracture risk; the large degree of overlap in bone mass values between subjects with, and without, fracture suggests that the combined sensitivity and specificity of screening would be relatively low but more prospective data are required, particularly for vertebral fracture. Secondly, treatment strategies based on different levels of bone mass have not been tested; such studies are required not only to indicate the efficacy of hormone replacement therapy in preventing fracture at different levels of bone mass but also to establish optimal duration of therapy and to assess compliance. Finally, there is insufficient knowledge at present to enable accurate estimation of the cost-effectiveness of screening programmes for osteoporosis. Some estimates, based solely on hip fracture, have been made but these are inevitably based on a number of assumptions, particularly with respect to compliance and the extra-skeletal risks and benefits of hormone replacement therapy. Furthermore, although hip fractures undoubtedly have a high morbidity and mortality they mostly occur in the very elderly; there is evidence that osteopenia in this age-group is associated with frailty and poor health so that prevention of hip fracture may not significantly prolong life and may merely divert the costs of hip fracture to those of other conditions, for example, stroke. Prevention of vertebral fracture may well be a more important target for a screening programme in view of the younger age at which these occur and their high morbidity; however, knowledge of the incidence and morbidity of these fractures is required before any estimate of cost-effectiveness can be made.

Biochemical indices of bone loss

Biochemical indices of bone turnover are described in Chapter 1; they include serum alkaline phosphatase and osteocalcin as markers of bone formation and serum tartrate-resistant acid phosphatase and urinary excretion of calcium, hydroxyproline and collagen cross-links as indices of resorption. These markers can provide valuable information about whole body rates of bone loss at the time of measurement, reflecting changes in bone turnover rather than in remodelling balance. They do not, however, indicate the level of bone mass from which loss occurred nor can it be assumed that rates of bone loss demonstrated at one point in time will be maintained over longer periods. Finally, they do not provide any information about the skeletal distribution of bone loss. For all these reasons, biochemical markers of bone turnover are unlikely to prove useful in screening for osteoporosis, although they can provide valuable information about the pathophysiology of bone loss in various conditions and may be useful in indicating short-term responsiveness to therapy.

Risk factors

In general, clinical and historical risk factors are only weakly predictive of bone mass and fracture risk and perform poorly as a screening method. Several studies in peri- and post-menopausal women have demonstrated that analysis of a variety of established and putative risk factors would reduce the necessity for bone mass assessent in a screening programme by only 25–30% and discriminates poorly between fracture and non-fracture cases. Risk factors for low bone mass probably differ between skeletal sites and are known to differ for different fracture types; for example, factors which affect the risk of falling and the associated neuromuscular protective responses are of paramount importance for hip fractures but much less so for vertebral fractures. The predictive value of risk factors is further weakened by their high prevalence in the population; in one study, it was estimated that 91% of middle-aged or elderly women in a population survey had four or more risk factors for osteoporosis.

Thus at present bone mass is the best available predictor of fracture risk although current evidence suggests that its combined sensitivity and specificity are insufficient to justify population screening. Whilst putative and established risk factors perform relatively poorly as predictors of bone mass or fracture risk they have an important role as diagnostic tools, particularly where bone densitometry is not readily available. High risk factors such as premature menopause, long-term, high dose corticosteroid therapy, low body weight and amenorrhoea, and a past history of fragility fracture can be regarded as an indication for treatment without the necessity for bone densitometry and more widespread recognition of these risk factors would undoubtedly lead to improved detection and prevention of osteoporosis. Weaker risk factors do not generally merit bone densitometry unless multiple.

Rare forms of osteoporosis

Idiopathic juvenile osteoporosis

Idiopathic juvenile osteoporosis is an extremely rare condition which occurs before the onset of puberty and is characterised by severe peripheral and spinal osteoporosis. The cause is unknown and the pathophysiology has not been defined. The disease typically presents in a previously healthy child with pains in the back, hips and legs and fractures may be seen in the spine and lower extremities. Deformities of the spine are common and include dorsal kyphosis, kyphoscoliosis and pigeon chest. Increased urinary excretion of hydroxyproline and hypercalcaemia have been described but in other cases no biochemical abnormalities are seen. Radiology reveals generalised osteopenia, vertebral deformity and the so-called neo-osseous osteoporosis, in which impaction-type fractures are

seen at sites of newly formed weight-bearing metaphyseal bone, particularly at the distal tibiae and adjacent to the knee and hip joints. The prognosis
is good in the majority of cases although, in a minority, deformities persist.
No specific treatment has been shown to be beneficial and since the
condition is generally reversible, emphasis should be placed on supportive
therapy with early mobilisation after fracture.

Regional osteoporosis

This condition, also known as transient or migratory osteoporosis,
algodystrophy, and Sudek's atrophy occurs most commonly after immobilisation but may also occur without any precipitating cause. Clinical
features include pain and swelling of an extremity, usually unilateral and
often associated with signs of autonomic instability. Radiological investigation shows patchy or diffuse demineralisation, particularly in the
subchondral region. Later there may be some atrophy of the subcutaneous
tissue, muscle wasting and radiological evidence of more severe osteopenia
in the affected region. In some cases, complete resolution occurs whilst, in
others, there are permanent sequelae; occasionally the disease shows a
migratory pattern. Treatment is mainly directed at early mobilisation of the
affected limb.

Osteoporosis of pregnancy

This is a rare and poorly understood condition in which severe osteoporosis
develops during the gestation and lactation period. Both the axial and
appendicular skeleton may be affected; hip involvement, sometimes with
spontaneous fracture is particularly characteristic but vertebral fractures
develop in some cases. The cause is unknown and the condition resolves
spontaneously over the course of some months in the majority of cases.
Subsequent pregnancies are not necessarily associated with a recurrence of
osteoporosis. No effective intervention has been defined.

Prevention and treatment of osteoporosis (Table 2.7)

General considerations

The clinical manifestations of osteoporosis appear after many years of
bone loss and by the time fracture occurs, irreversible loss of bone mass and
structure are likely to have occurred. Treatment of established osteoporosis

Table. 2.7. *Agents used in the prevention and*
treatment of osteoporosis

Agent
Hormone replacement therapy
Bisphosphonates
Calcitonin
Sodium fluoride
Anabolic steroids
Vitamin D
Calcium

is thus often unsatisfactory for both patient and physician, whereas effective prevention can often be achieved.

Most of the measures adopted in the treatment of established osteoporosis are also likely to be effective in its prevention. The importance of early detection of disease and institution of prophylactic therapy cannot be overemphasised; however, despite the considerable advances in this area, treatment of established osteoporosis presents an increasingly common problem for many physicians and general practitioners. Whereas the major target of prophylactic measures is to prevent fracture, the aim of treatment in patients with established disease is both to reduce the risk of further fracture and to alleviate existing symptoms. The pain associated with vertebral fractures is often underestimated and its treatment correspondingly inadequate; appropriate analgesic therapy in the early stages not only provides symptomatic relief but also ensures that immobility following the fracture, which may further compromise bone mass, is reduced to a minimum. Unfortunately, in some patients, severe pain persists for months or even years and in such cases some compromise in the degree of pain reduction is often necessary to avoid side-effects or dependence. In many cases, poor posture and paravertebral muscle spasm contribute to pain and these may benefit from physiotherapy. Spinal supports, in the form of surgical corsets, are not recommended because they produce a relative immobilisation of the spine which is likely to have adverse effects on bone mass.

The psycho-social effects of osteoporosis may be devastating to the patient; whilst many of the long-term consequences of the disease, such as spinal deformity and height loss cannot be reversed, supportive therapy plays an important role. Physiotherapy may help postural abnormalities associated with spinal deformity and advice should be given about avoidance of trauma which might precipitate further fractures, while emphasising the importance of appropriate physical activity. Patient education about the disease is often constructive and may provide reassurance to those with loss of confidence associated with spinal deformity and past fracture.

Hormone replacement therapy

Hormone replacement therapy is unique in its proven ability to reduce fracture risk both in the spine and hip and is used both in the prevention and treatment of osteoporosis. Hormone replacement during and after the menopause prevents menopausal bone loss and may even increase bone mass. The degree of protection afforded against fractures is uncertain; retrospective data indicate an overall reduction in hip fracture risk of 50–75% but these studies are biased by the likelihood that women using hormone replacement therapy are intrinsically healthier than non-users, so the magnitude of protection may be overestimated.

Despite the undoubted benefits of hormone replacement therapy, both for bone mass and fracture risk, some important aspects of treatment remain ill defined. Whilst there is general agreement that treatment should be started as early as possible in the menopause, the optimum duration of therapy is unclear. It has been claimed by some that once hormone replacement therapy is stopped, subsequent bone loss is accelerated and within a few years all benefits of treatment on bone mass have been lost; if true, the implication of this is that only life-long hormone replacement therapy would only be effective. Other data suggest that a finite period of hormone replacement 'buys time' for the skeleton and that bone loss after cessation of therapy occurs at the normal rate but from a higher level of bone mass, so at any given post-menopausal age bone mass will be higher than if therapy had not been given. Resolution of this controversy requires further information on patterns of bone loss following cessation of therapy; because of fears about increased risk of breast cancer after 5–10 years of hormone replacement therapy, many physicians advise treatment for around five years but revision of this policy may be indicated as further information emerges.

Formulations and dosage of hormone replacement therapy

A number of preparations, involving a variety of oestrogenic and progestagenic compounds and different modes of administration, are available for use as hormone replacement therapy and the choice is likely to

Table. 2.8. *Unopposed oestrogen replacement therapy*

Product	Composition (daily dose)
Harmogen®	Piperazine oestrone sulphate (1.5 mg)
Premarin®	Conjugated equine oestrogens (0.625 or 1.25 mg)
Climaval®	Oestradiol valerate (1 or 2 mg)
Hormonin®	Oestriol (0.27 mg) + oestrone (1.4 mg) + oestradiol (0.6 mg)

increase further in the near future (Tables 2.8 and 2.9). Because of the increased risk of endometrial cancer in women receiving unopposed oestrogens, combined oestrogen/progestagen therapy is generally indicated in women with an intact uterus although, as discussed below, there may be exceptions to this rule. The choice of preparation is dictated mainly by cost, patient preference and, in some cases, medical considerations; issues of safety and efficacy are not sufficiently well defined to influence decisions about particular regimes. Although the majority of evidence for benefits on bone mass and fracture risk have been obtained using unopposed oestrogens, combined preparations appear to have similar effects and some progestagens have been shown independently to reduce menopausal bone loss.

Oestrogen preparations

Oestrogens may be administered orally, parenterally or transdermally; the beneficial effects on bone mass appear to be quantitatively similar for all these routes, although reduction in fracture risk has only been demonstrated using oral oestrogens. The degree of systemic absorption from vaginal oestrogen preparations is variable, and there is no evidence that this form of administration protects the skeleton. Whereas synthetic oestrogens are used in oral contraceptives, nearly all hormone replacement preparations contain natural oestrogens, which are 100–1000 times less potent and do not confer protection against conception. Oral oestrogens are most widely used although transdermal preparations are becoming increasingly popular. Because of the hepatic first-pass effect, most of the oestrogen is converted to oestrone and relatively high doses are therefore required, producing high peak concentrations which may sometimes give rise to side-effects such as nausea or dyspepsia. Nevertheless, oral preparations are generally well tolerated and effective in preventing bone loss and alleviating menopausal symptoms.

Transdermal or parenteral oestrogens are specifically indicated in

Table. 2.9. *Combined hormone replacement therapy preparations*

Product	Mode of administration	Oestrogen (daily dose)	Progestagen (daily dose) 10–14	Cyclical/continuous (oestrogen)
Prempak–C®	Oral	Conjugated equine oestrogens (0.625 or 1.25 mg)	Norgestrel (0.15 mg)	Continuous
Trisequens®	Oral	Oestradiol (1.2 mg) Oestriol (0.5–1 mg)	Norethisterone acetate (1 mg)	Continuous
Cycloprogynova®	Oral	Oestradiol valerate (1 or 2 mg)	Levonorgestrel (0.25 mg)	Cyclical
Estrapak®	Transdermal (oestrogen) + oral (progestagen)	Oestradiol (50 µg)	Norethisterone acetate (1 mg)	Continuous
Estracombi®	Transdermal	Oestradiol (50 µg)	Norethisterone acetate (250 µg)	Continuous

women with malabsorption or liver disease; they should also be used in the minority of women who cannot tolerate oral oestrogens, since symptoms such as nausea and breast tenderness appear to be less common with non-oral preparations. However, skin reactions to transdermal oestrogens occur in 25–30% of cases, usually in the form of mild erythema. In a small percentage of cases, blistering occurs and is sufficiently severe to necessitate withdrawal of treatment. Poor adhesion of the patches, which are changed twice weekly, may also present problems. In women with an intact uterus, progestagens should be given orally for 10–12 days of each cycle. Subcutaneous oestradiol implants avoid problems of poor compliance but the plasma levels of oestradiol produced vary considerably and high levels in some cases lead to unacceptable side-effects. Tachyphylaxis has been described in some patients, with recurrence of menopausal symptoms despite apparently adequate plasma oestradiol levels; such patients request implants at increasingly short time intervals. In general, oestradiol implants should be replaced at six to nine monthly intervals and, as with transdermal oestrogens, a progestagen must be administered for 10–12 days of each cycle in women with an intact uterus.

Progestagen preparations

Progestagens protect the endometrium from oestrogen-induced hyperplasia and carcinoma and should be given to all non-hysterectomised women receiving hormone replacement unless specific contraindications exist. The progestagen should be given for 10–12 days each month and is nearly always administered orally, although rectal, vaginal or parenteral preparations are available if absorption of oral preparations is inadequate and transdermal delivery of norethisterone acetate is now possible. Commonly used progestagens are either derivatives of nortestosterone (norethisterone, levonorgestrel) or are derived from progesterone itself (dydrogesterone, medroxyprogesterone acetate) (Table 2.8). More recently, gestogene, desogestrel and norgestimate, which are derivatives of levonorgestrel have been developed.

Side-effects of hormone replacement therapy (Table 2.10)

Oestrogens

Side-effects attributable to oestrogen therapy are most common in the first few months of treatment and include nausea, breast and nipple tenderness and, less commonly, epigastric discomfort; these symptoms are more

Table. 2.10. *Side effects of hormone replacement therapy*

	Oestrogen	Progestagen
Short-term:	Nausea	Breast tenderness
	Breast tenderness	Oedema
	Epigastric discomfort	Nausea
	Vaginal bleeding	Mood changes
		Androgenic effects
Long term:	Endometrial cancer (if unopposed) ?Breast cancer	?Cardiovascular disease

common in women who start treatment some years after the menopause. In a minority of cases, side-effects persist and reduction of the dose should be considered. Alternatively, relief of symptoms may sometimes be achieved by using a different oral preparation or by changing to transdermal administration.

From the patient's point of view, the occurrence of monthly withdrawal bleeding is often the most troublesome consequence of oestrogen therapy. Continuous administration of progestagen and oestrogen results in amenorrhoea in the majority of patients, but the high incidence of irregular bleeding, particularly in the first six months of treatment and side-effects attributable to the progestagen reduce compliance with this regime. Tibolone, a synthetic steroid with oestrogenic, androgenic and progestagenic properties is now available for the treatment of menopausal symptoms, and has been shown to prevent bone loss in the radius, femur and spine. It is given continuously and when administered one or more years post-menopausally does not cause vaginal bleeding in the majority of women; it is most likely to cause bleeding in women who are peri-menopausal and thus should not be prescribed within one year of the last natural menstrual period. Because relatively few data are available on its ability to prevent bone loss and its effect on fracture risk has not been documented, its use in the prevention and treatment of osteoporosis should be reserved for those women who will not tolerate withdrawal bleeding. Symptoms attributable to the progestagenic component of tibolone (see below) may occur in women who are progestagen-sensitive.

Progestagens

Progestagen therapy may cause breast tenderness, oedema, abdominal bloating and nausea. Psychological complaints also occur and include depression, anxiety and lability of mood. Side-effects due to progestagen tend to be more common and more severe than those attributable to oestrogen therapy and are an important cause of non-compliance with combined hormone replacement therapy.

Long-term risks and benefits of hormone replacement therapy

Cardiovascular disease

The risks and benefits of long-term, combined hormone replacement are unknown. Present knowledge is almost entirely derived from studies, mainly retrospective, of women taking unopposed oestrogens; these have mostly shown a substantial protection against ischaemic heart disease and, less certainly, stroke. The reduction in ischaemic heart disease reported in menopausal oestrogen users is of the order of 50%; the magnitude of this effect may have been overestimated by observational studies because of their failure accurately to correct for possible intrinsic and confounding differences between oestrogen users and non-users.

The mechanism by which this protection occurs is poorly understood but may be related to oestrogen-induced changes in lipoprotein profile, glucose metabolism, coagulation, fibrinolysis and blood pressure. The effect of added progestagen therapy on the cardiovascular protection conferred by oestrogens is unknown. At least some of the progestagens currently used in hormone replacement therapy formulations have adverse effects on blood lipoprotein levels, decreasing high density lipoprotein (HDL) cholesterol levels and increasing low density lipoprotein (LDL) cholesterol; these effects are most marked with the androgenic progestagens. Whether these changes affect the cardiovascular benefits conferred by unopposed oestrogens is unknown. However, in women at high risk from ischaemic heart disease, there is a case to be made for treatment with unopposed oestrogens even when the uterus is intact, providing that endometrial biopsies are performed at yearly intervals or earlier if irregular bleeding occurs. The alternative is to use a progestagen which does not adversely affect lipids, for example medroxyprogesterone.

Breast cancer

There is now considerable evidence that oestrogen therapy for longer than five or so years increases the risk of breast cancer in postmenopausal women. The magnitude of this increase in risk is uncertain as is the exact point in time at which risk begins to increase, but current opinion is that treatment for five years or less is not associated with any appreciable

Table. 2.11. *Contraindications to hormone replacement therapy*

Absolute	Relative
Breast cancer	Endometriosis
Endometrial cancer	Venous thromboembolic disease
Malignant melanoma	Hypertension
Undiagnosed vaginal bleeding	Fibroids
	Active liver disease
	Gallstones

increase in incidence. The risk appears to be greater with high dose preparations but the question of whether it varies with different kinds of oestrogen (i.e. synthetic or natural) or with different modes of administration has not been resolved. It is also unclear whether the addition of a progestagen affects this risk.

The possibility that hormone replacement therapy may increase breast cancer risk makes some women understandably reluctant to embark on long-term treatment. This risk has to be weighed up against that of osteoporotic fracture; if the latter is high, many women will be persuaded that the benefits of treatment will outweigh any increase in breast cancer risk. The issue of duration of therapy has been discussed earlier. Whilst the data on breast cancer risk suggest that treatment for five years or less will not increase breast cancer risk, concern has been expressed that this duration of therapy will be ineffective in preventing hip fracture.

Contraindications to hormone replacement therapy (Table 2.11)

The only absolute contraindications to hormone replacement therapy are breast cancer, endometrial cancer, malignant melanoma and pregnancy; in addition, hormone replacement should not be given to women with vaginal bleeding of unknown cause. Relative contraindications are shown in Table 2.9. In women with chronic liver disease, non-oral preparations should be prescribed. There is no evidence that hormone replacement increases the risk of spontaneous venous thrombosis in women with a past history, although some studies have demonstrated adverse effects of oral preparations on fibrinolysis and coagulation. Since non-oral formulations do not appear to have these effects, their use may be preferable in women with a significant clinical history of venous thromboembolic disease. Although hypertension develops in a small percentage of women taking hormone replacement therapy, it can be controlled by antihypertensive drugs and does not usually require permanent withdrawal of hormone therapy. Endometriosis may be reactivated by hormone replacement therapy, even many years after the menopause and may necessitate withdrawal of treatment; women with a history of this condition should be warned about the possibility of recurrence of symptoms. Hormone replacement therapy may also lead to an increase in the size of fibroids; if there are strong indications for hormone replacement, hysterectomy may be considered if symptoms recur. Oral hormone replacement increases the lithogenicity of bile and may exacerbate gallstone disease; it is likely but unproven that non-oral preparations may have less adverse effects on bile composition. A past history of endometrial hyperplasia, with the exception of severe atypical forms, is not a contraindication to hormone replacement therapy although endometrial biopsy should be carried out after around six months of treatment.

A past or present history of ischaemic heart disease is often quoted as a contraindication to hormone replacement therapy but there is no evidence to support this view. Indeed, the protective effect of oestrogens in this respect has led some to advocate that hormone replacement should be universally recommended to postmenopausal women. The possibility that progestagens may reduce or even reverse the beneficial effects of oestrogens raises the question of whether, in high risk women, unopposed therapy should be given even when the uterus is intact. The much higher morbidity and mortality of coronary heart disease compared to endometrial cancer argues strongly for this approach; in such cases endometrial biopsies should be performed at yearly intervals or sooner if irregular bleeding occurs.

Follow-up of women taking long-term hormone replacement therapy

There are no universally agreed recommendations for the follow-up of women on long-term hormone replacement therapy. It is important that access to professional advice is available for women who develop irregular vaginal bleeding and that women are aware of the need to seek medical advice under these circumstances. Endometrial biopsies for women on combined therapy are not indicated unless abnormal bleeding patterns occur, nor is there any need to increase the frequency of cervical smears. Mammography should be performed as currently recommended for all UK women over the age of 50 years; current evidence indicates that there is no reason to increase the frequency of examination or to reduce the lower age limit in women receiving long-term hormone replacement therapy.

The majority of women taking hormone replacement therapy are well and asymptomatic and yearly visits to their general practitioner are adequate. Although some doctors perform breast and pelvic examinations every one to two years there is no evidence that this practice confers any benefit. The availability of bone densitometry is insufficient to enable routine follow-up measurements; these are unnecessary in the majority of women but may be valuable in detecting those who fail to respond due to lack of compliance or other factors, for example malabsorption or corticosteroid therapy.

Indications for long-term hormone replacement therapy

In the majority of women, the decision about whether or not to take hormone replacement therapy is based on the presence or absence of menopausal symptoms. When used for this purpose, the duration of treatment is generally less than two years, whereas prevention of osteoporosis probably requires at least five years' continuous therapy.

Well-defined indications for long-term hormone replacement therapy include established osteoporosis (the presence of one or more spinal or peripheral fragility fractures) in women aged 70 years or less, premature menopause (before the age of 40 years), and prolonged secondary amenorrhoea associated with conditions such as Crohn's disease and anorexia nervosa. The belief that hormone replacement therapy should be restricted to peri-menopausal women is no longer held; there is evidence that it has beneficial effects on bone mass up to the age of at least 70 years. Densitometric criteria for long-term hormone replacement therapy are much less clear. Some favour treatment if bone mass at the menopause is less than one standard deviation below the mean value for normal pre-menopausal women, whilst others use different criteria based on the reference range for age-matched women. Until different treatment protocols have been formally tested, the level of bone mass at which treatment should be advised remains a matter of conjecture. In the absence of absolute indications, decisions about long-term hormone replacement therapy are usually made by both the physician and patient, and take into account a number of factors, of which bone density is only one.

Bisphosphonates

Over the last few years there has been increasing interest in the use of bisphosphonates for the treatment of osteoporosis. These drugs primarily

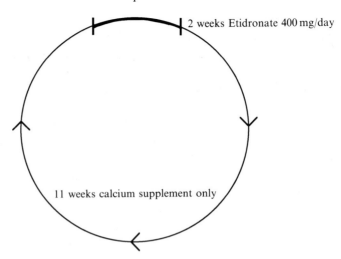

Fig. 2.5. Regime used for etidronate therapy in the treatment of osteoporosis.

act by inhibiting bone resorption although they may also have an anabolic effect on bone.

Two trials of the first generation bisphosphonate, etidronate, have recently been reported in post-menopausal women with established osteoporosis. In both these studies, the drug was given intermittently, the rationale being that bisphosphonates have a long half-life in bone and also that this mode of administration should prevent adverse effects on bone mineralisation. The primary end-point of both studies was to investigate the effect of intermittent etidronate/calcium therapy on bone mass and impressive benefits were demonstrated, a 20% increase in lumbar spine density being shown in one study after 5 years. Smaller, but positive, effects on cortical bone mass were also seen. A significant reduction in vertebral fracture rate was reported after three years' treatment although subsequent data from these studies have indicated that their design precludes definite conclusions to be drawn about effects of the regime on fracture rate. Nevertheless, the documented effects on spinal bone mass are encouraging and suggest that beneficial effects on spinal fracture rate may well occur. It should be noted that there are no data concerning the effects of bisphosphonates on hip fracture risk.

The regime currently used in the UK (Didronel PMO) consists of repeated cycles of a two-week course of etidronate, 400 mg nocte, followed by 11 weeks of calcium citrate, 500 mg/day (Fig. 2.5). Because gastrointestinal absorption of etidronate is poor, the bisphosphonate should be taken at least two hours clear of meals and is thus best taken last thing at night.

Concurrent intake of calcium supplements further reduces the absorption, and for this reason calcium is omitted during the two-week courses of etidronate. The effects of various regimes of newer bisphosphonates, for example pamidronate, clodronate and tiludronate, are now under investigation, both for the prevention of menopausal bone loss and the treatment of established osteoporosis.

Bisphosphonates thus represent an exciting new possibility for the prevention and treatment of osteoporosis, but more information is required before their therapeutic role becomes established. At present, they provide an alternative for post-menopausal osteoporosis in women who are unable or unwilling to tolerate hormone replacement therapy. Their role in the prevention of menopausal bone loss and in treatment of osteoporosis in men remains to be defined.

Bisphosphonates are safe and have few side-effects. Nausea and diarrhoea occur in a small percentage, but adverse effects on bone mineralisation, sometimes seen with the higher doses used for the treatment of Paget's disease, have not been encountered with the cyclical, intermittent etidronate regime used for osteoporosis.

Sodium fluoride

Sodium fluoride is a potent stimulator of bone formation which acts by increasing the proliferative capacity of osteoblastic cells, leading to an increase in bone formation rate at both tissue and cellular level. Although the ability of sodium fluoride to increase trabecular bone mass in the axial skeleton is well established, its role in the treatment of osteoporosis is controversial. In two American studies, an average daily dose of 75 mg for five years was not associated with any reduction in vertebral fracture rate in women with post-menopausal osteoporosis; however, in another study from France, patients treated with 50 mg of sodium fluoride for two years were significantly less likely to develop a new vertebral fracture than patients treated with other regimes which did not include sodium fluoride. Moreover, when data from the largest American study were reanalysed to take different dosages into account, it became apparent that doses of around 50 mg/day were associated with a reduction in fracture rate.

Both the therapeutic effects and the side-effects of sodium fluoride are closely dose related, with a narrow 'therapeutic window.' Low doses produce insufficient osteoblastic stimulation for clinically significant improvements in bone mass to occur whilst high doses are associated with a high incidence of gastro-intestinal and musculo-skeletal side-effects and the formation of abnormal, mechanically inferior, bone. There is also some concern that the increase in trabecular bone mass may occur at the expense of cortical bone; a reduction in cortical bone mass has been reported in some studies whereas others have not shown any loss. An increased incidence of non-vertebral fractures has been reported in some studies after treatment with doses of 50 mg/day or more of sodium fluoride, possibly attributable to the formation of abnormal, mechanically weak bone and/or adverse effects on cortical bone mass. Both complete and incomplete fractures have been described; the latter, which resemble stress fractures, occur predominantly in weight-bearing bones and form part of the 'lower extremity pain syndrome' (LEPS) which is dose-related and occurs in 15–35% of treated patients.

The therapeutic role of sodium fluoride thus remains to be clearly defined. Its potent anabolic effects suggest that it may have considerable potential as a therapeutic agent for established osteoporosis but the dose used is critical and requirements may vary between patients, depending on factors such as gastro-intestinal absorption and bioavailability of the formulation used. In this respect, measurement of circulating fluoride concentrations may be of value in determining the optimal dose. Bone mass, both in the spine and the femur, should be carefully monitored in patients treated with sodium fluoride to detect those with low femoral bone mass who may be at increased risk of hip fracture and to identify the minority who fail to respond. Calcium supplements, at a dose of 1000 mg elemental calcium daily, should be given to all patients receiving sodium fluoride and bone biopsy should be performed after two to three years' treatment to detect mineralisation defects, which may occur in some patients. The recommended dose is between 40 and 60 mg daily and treatment should not exceed five years.

Calcitonin

Calcitonin inhibits bone resorption and has been shown to reduce or prevent menopausal bone loss in the spine, although its effects on cortical bone loss are less certain and there is no evidence that it reduces fracture rate. At present, only parenteral formulations of calcitonin are generally available in the UK; however, intra-nasal preparations are being developed and may be in use in the near future.

Calcitonin has significant analgesic properties and is often effective in the treatment of bone pain associated with vertebral fracture, particularly in its acute phase. Salmon calcitonin is generally used and is given at a dose of

100 IU daily for some weeks until symptomatic relief has been obtained. The treatment may be repeated if necessary.

Side-effects are not infrequent with parenteral calcitonin and include nausea, vomiting, flushing, tingling of the hands and an unpleasant taste in the mouth.

Anabolic steroids

Stanozolol and nandrolone decanoate are synthetic derivatives of natural androgens which have been shown to reduce the rate of bone loss in osteoporosis. Administration of these agents to patients with established osteoporosis results in small increases in axial and appendicular bone mass, but the effects on fracture rate at any site are unknown. Stanozolol is given orally in a dose of 5 mg daily, whereas nandrolone is administered intramuscularly in a dose of 50 mg every three to four weeks.

Adverse effects are relatively common and include androgenic manifestations such as hirsutism and hoarseness and lowering of the voice. Salt and water retention may lead to oedema and increases in hepatic transaminases may occur, the latter being more common with stanozolol. Skin rashes, dyspepsia, muscle cramps and headache may also occur.

Parathyroid hormone

Low doses of synthetic parathyroid hormone fragments (the first 34–38 amino acids) have anabolic effects on bone and lead to an increase in axial trabecular bone mass in patients with established spinal osteoporosis. The peptide is administered intramuscularly. There are no data on the effect of such treatment on fracture rate, and the role of this therapy in the treatment of osteoporosis remains to be defined.

Calcium

The case for, and against, calcium supplementation in the prevention and treatment of osteoporosis has been argued vigorously over the years. Intestinal absorption of calcium decreases with age and a negative calcium balance can be demonstrated in the majority of post-menopausal women. There is now good evidence that calcium supplementation reduces both trabecular and cortical bone loss although a protective effect against fracture has not been definitively demonstrated; calcium should not be regarded as a substitute for hormone replacement or other therapy but

Table. 2.12. *Calcium content of some foods*

Product	Quantity	mg calcium
Cheddar cheese	100 g	800
Cottage cheese	100 g	60
Milk (semi-skimmed)	1 pint	729
Milk (full cream)	1 pint	702
Butter	100 g	15
Yoghurt	125 g	225
Milk chocolate	100 g	220
Muesli	55 g	110
White bread	1 slice	55
Wholemeal bread	1 slice	13
Canned sardines in oil	100 g	550
Canned pilchards in oil	100 g	300
Haddock (steamed or poached)	100 g	55
Broccoli (raw)	100 g	100
Spring greens	100 g	86
Baked beans	100 g	45
Spinach (fresh)	100 g	130
Dried figs	100 g	280

Table. 2.13. *Calcium supplements suitable for use in the prevention or treatment of osteoporosis*

Product	Form	mg calcium/tablet or pack
Cacit®	Effervescent tablet	500
Calcichew®	Chewable tablet	500
Calcidrink®	Granules	1000
Calcium-500	Tablet	500
Citrical®	Granules	500
Sandocal-400®	Effervescent tablet	400
Sandocal-1000®	Effervescent tablet	1000
Ossopan®	Granules	712

rather as an adjunct to treatment. A daily calcium intake of between 1000 and 1500 mg daily is believed to be necessary to maintain calcium balance in peri- and post-menopausal women; in some cases, this may be achieved through dietary intake (Table 2.12) but in those who are unable to ingest adequate amounts of dairy produce, calcium supplements should be advised, since much of the calcium present in green vegetables is not bioavailable. A daily dose of 1000 to 1500 mg of elemental calcium (Table 2.13), taken with meals and preferably in divided doses should be prescribed; the dose should be tailored according to dietary intake. In the absence of hypercalcaemia or renal stone disease such doses are safe and free from side-effects.

Physical exercise

Weight-bearing exercise results in an increase in bone mass at the loaded site whilst immobilisation leads to rapid bone loss. The role, however, of physical exercise in the prevention or treatment of osteoporosis remains uncertain. Physical exercise is generally beneficial for all age-groups and, in the elderly, the resulting increase in physical fitness may reduce the likelihood of falls and improve the protective neuromuscular responses associated with falling. In post-menopausal women there is evidence that weight-bearing exercise may have small mitigating effects on menopausal bone loss but, as with calcium, exercise should not be regarded as a definitive treatment in these women. In patients with established osteoporosis gentle exercise may improve mobility, well-being and posture, but the effects on bone mass and fracture risk are unknown. Finally, it should be noted that extreme exercise in young women may have adverse effects on bone mass because of the development of oestrogen deficiency and amenorrhoea in some cases.

Vitamin D

The role of vitamin D in the prevention and treatment of osteoporosis is currently a topic of considerable interest. In elderly subjects, in whom subclinical vitamin D deficiency and secondary hyperparathyroidism are relatively common in the UK and some other European countries, vitamin D supplementation may reduce age-related bone loss; evidence from France indicates that this approach may also reduce hip fracture risk in the elderly population. Small doses of vitamin D (400 IU daily) have also been shown to have beneficial effects on spinal bone mass in healthy post-menopausal women. In women with post-menopausal osteoporosis, calcitriol (1,25-dihydroxyvitamin D), in doses of 0.5–1.0 µg/day prevents bone loss and increases trabecular and cortical bone mass; recent data suggest that this treatment may also reduce vertebral fracture risk. However, active vitamin D metabolites must be used with caution, particularly in the elderly, because of the risk of hypercalcaemia, hypercalciuria and renal damage.

Summary

Hormone replacement therapy is the current regime of choice for the prevention and treatment of osteoporosis in peri- and post-menopausal women and in pre-menopausal women with prolonged secondary amenorrhoea. Bisphosphonates or calcitonin provide alternative approaches to the prevention of osteoporosis in women for whom hormone replacement is contraindicated, although their effects on fracture risk, particularly in the hip, are less well documented. For the treatment of established osteoporosis in men, and in women in whom hormone replacement therapy cannot be used, options include bisphosphonates, sodium fluoride, calcitonin and anabolic steroids. Vitamin D supplements may be beneficial in the elderly and active vitamin D metabolites may also have a role in the treatment of post-menopausal osteoporosis. Avoidance of known risk factors should be encouraged, and an appropriate level of physical activity maintained. A daily calcium intake of at least 1000 mg should be ensured, either through dietary means or with the use of calcium supplements.

Hormone replacement, bisphosphonate, and calcium therapy require relatively little monitoring and are ideal for use in general practice. Calcitonin is safe but the present unavailability of non-parenteral preparations limits its use. Other forms of treatment, particularly sodium fluoride, require careful supervision both from the point of view of uncertainty about therapeutic efficacy and because of potentially serious adverse effects. The treatment of secondary osteoporosis should be directed, where possible, towards management of the underlying cause. The effects of hormone replacement therapy in women with steroid-induced osteoporosis have not been conclusively demonstrated but many believe that hormone replacement should be given routinely to peri-menopausal women on long-term steroids. There is evidence that bisphosphonates prevent steroid-induced bone loss but the regime currently available on prescription in the UK (Didronel PMO) has not been evaluated.

Further reading

Compston, J.E. (1990). Osteoporosis. *Clinical Endocrinology*, **33**, 653–82.
Khaw, K.T. (ed.) (1992). Hormone replacement therapy. *British Medical Bulletin*, **48**(2), 249–476.
Melton, L.J., Eddy, D.M. & Johnston, C.C. (1990). Screening for osteoporosis. *Annals of Internal Medicine*, **112**, 516–28.
Reid, I.R. (1989). Pathogenesis and treatment of steroid-induced osteoporosis. *Clinical Science*, **30**, 83–103.
Riggs, B.L. & Melton, J. (1986). Involutional osteoporosis. *New England Journal of Medicine*, **314**, 1676–86.

3

Osteomalacia

Osteomalacia, meaning soft bones, was first recognised as a separate entity from osteoporosis by the German pathologist Pommer in 1885. It is a condition in which there is a failure of bone mineralisation usually resulting histologically in an excess of poorly calcified osteoid bone matrix. In rickets, in children, there is an additional defective mineralisation of cartilage, and in particular of the epiphyseal growth plates.

The clinical importance of the condition lies in the skeletal deformities and manifestations of hypocalcaemia produced in early life and the muscle weakness, bone pain and fractures seen in adults. The main causes (Table 3.1) can be summarised as either due to a deficiency of Vitamin D and its metabolites or due to resistance to the vitamin. The cause of osteomalacia in developed countries is mainly confined to those affected by Vitamin D deficiency, and therefore the majority of this chapter is devoted to the management of these groups of patients, although some of the other rarer causes are discussed for information.

Vitamin D deficiency

This privational form of osteomalacia is mainly associated with young adults in the Asian community and with the elderly in the general population. In the Asian community, the disease mainly affects young women and girls during the pubertal spurt in bone growth. The prevalence in the elderly population is not known, but studies on unselected acute admissions to geriatric units in the UK suggest a figure of 4% in those admissions.

Risk factors and vitamin D metabolism

Vitamin D metabolism is summarised in Fig. 3.1. Vitamin D was so named because it was discovered after Vitamins A, B and C had been identified.

Table. 3.1. *Causes of Osteomalacia*

Vitamin D deficiency	Lack of sunlight
	Poor nutrition
	Malabsorption syndrome
Impaired hydroxylation of parent Vitamin D to active metabolites	Chronic renal failure
	Tumour induced
	Vitamin D dependent rickets Type I
End organ resistance to 1:25 $(OH)_2$ Vitamin D	Vitamin D dependent rickets Type II
Hypophosphataemic states	Inherited hypophosphataemia
	Tumour induced
	Fanconi syndrome
Bone poisons	Aluminium
	Bisphosphonates
	Fluoride
Miscellaneous	Chronic metabolic acidosis
	Long-term haemodialysis
	Chronic parenteral nutrition

The term was used to describe the anti-rachitic substance in cod liver oil found to cure childhood rickets.

Most osteomalacia is multifactorial in origin, and a high clinical suspicion is necessary to avoid missing diagnosing the disease. The risk factors are summarised in Fig. 3.2.

Sunlight exposure

The major source of Vitamin D is from UV light from the sun with a wavelength of between 290 and 320μ converting 7-dehydrocholesterol found in the Malpighian layer of the skin to cholecalciferol. These wavelengths are filtered out by the atmosphere in the Autumn and Winter in the UK, as the sun does not rise high enough in the sky. There is therefore a seasonal variation in the incidence of the disease with peak incidence in the early Spring.

Atmospheric pollution will also filter out these wavelengths of UV light, and rickets was probably the first disease ascribed to industrial pollution when there was an epidemic amongst children of city factory workers during the Industrial Revolution in Europe. Autopsy studies suggested an 80–90% prevalence amongst children in some areas. It was subsequently discovered, in the late 1800s, that a Summer in the country would cure the

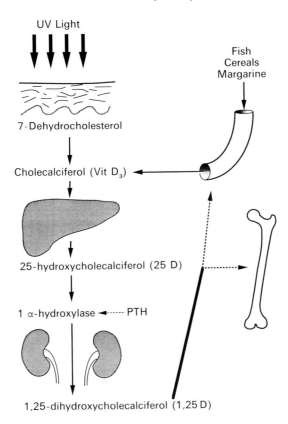

Fig. 3.1. Sources, activation and sites of action of Vitamin D.

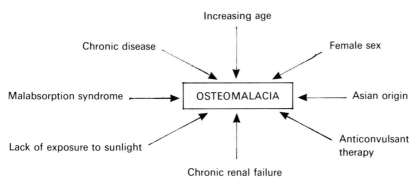

Fig. 3.2. Risk factors in the development of osteomalacia.

children, and for many years it was debated whether this effect was due to the sunlight or to the fresh air!

Avid seekers after a suntan do not get Vitamin D toxic because, in those circumstances, 7-dehydrocholesterol gets converted to the biologically inert lumisterol and tachysterol which are not removed from the skin, and are then sloughed off. The cholecalciferol however is removed by a specific Vitamin D-binding protein in the blood and stored predominantly in fat reserves.

Melanin absorbs UV light, so black skinned and more mildly pigmented people of Indian and Pakistani extraction require greater exposure to UV light than Caucasians to produce a similar amount of Vitamin D. However, the British West Indian population is free of clinical rickets compared with the less pigmented, yet more seriously affected, Asian community. Skin pigmentation, in isolation, therefore appears only to be a small risk factor.

Age

The reasons for osteomalacia being more common in older people are probably multifactorial. They include decreased sunlight exposure secondary to disability, poor diet and age-related decrease in the ability to control the hydroxylation of parent Vitamin D to the active metabolite. The cause of the increased female incidence is unknown. Serum levels of 25-hydroxy vitamin D do tend to decrease with age even in the healthy elderly, although the change is more pronounced in old people in hospital. Although ageing does appear to decrease the capacity of the skin to produce Vitamin D, there is such spare capacity for synthesis that, provided there is adequate sunlight exposure, ageing skin is unlikely to be involved in the production of a deficiency state. A relationship between decreasing levels of mobility and the presence of low 25-hydroxyvitamin D levels (<25 nmol/1) has been noted, and low levels are also far more common in the elderly who are housebound. This suggests that the major factor involved in the low 25-hydroxyvitamin D levels often found in old people is lack of exposure to sunlight. In these circumstances, dietary intake of Vitamin D becomes the major determinant of 25-hydroxyvitamin D levels. This hypothesis has been confirmed whereas there is no relationship between dietary intake of vitamin D and 25-hydroxyvitamin D levels in healthy individuals, a strong relationship does exist in sick old people. Other suggested mechanisms which may contribute in some patients include gastrointestinal malabsorption of Vitamin D (which has been observed in sick old people) and impaired hepatic hydroxylation.

Diet

Diet is a poor source of Vitamin D as, apart from fortified foods (such as cereals in the USA and UK and milk in the US), most foodstuffs contain minimal amounts. To achieve the recommended daily intake, one would have to consume eight eggs, 500 g of butter or 500 g of liver a day! Vitamin D is fat soluble and thus oily fish, e.g. sardines, mackerel, tuna and salmon is the only foodstuff to naturally contain large quantities of the vitamin.

Dietary intake, however, probably plays an important role in those groups who are at risk of osteomalacia on account of poor exposure to sunlight. For example, Asian women, who are particularly vulnerable, often extensively cover their skin and may only rarely venture outside, which, coupled with the effect of skin pigmentation, results in a near total dependancy on dietary intake. This may be also be insufficient as certain diets, such as the high fibre, low meat intake diets practised by many Hindus and Sikhs do appear to increase Vitamin D requirements. Mechanisms, which are probably multiple, include decreased calcium availability secondary to phytates binding dietary calcium and the interruption of the enterohepatic recirculation of Vitamin D metabolites by constituents of cereals, e.g. lignin.

Malabsorption syndromes

Osteomalacia has been frequently described in association with fat malabsorption states, especially following gastric surgery, as well as in many chronic small bowel, pancreatic and liver disorders. The most common disorders causing malabsorption associated with osteomalacia are post-gastrectomy, in Crohn's disease and in coeliac disease. In the latter condition, if untreated, prevalence rates of up to 50% have been described. Various mechanisms have been postulated. They include (i) impaired absorption of parent Vitamin D, (ii) the loss of the 20–30% of the circulating 25-hydroxyvitamin D involved in enterohepatic circulation, (iii) both a direct effect of fat malabsorption on calcium absorption itself, and an indirect effect if there is associated magnesium depletion, (iv) the avoidance of the outdoors and thus sunlight by patients with chronic illness.

Clinical features of vitamin D deficiency: osteomalacia and rickets

The clinical presentation of osteomalacia may differ according to the aetiology as well as the age at presentation of the disease. The most

common form, however, presenting to a general physician will be
osteomalacia secondary to Vitamin D deficiency, and it is therefore the
presentation described here unless other stated. The specific clinical
features of the other types of osteomalacia are described under their
individual entries. Acquired osteomalacia however is frequently multifactorial in origin and the symptoms may not neatly fit exactly into any one
classification.

The classical symptoms in adults consist of bone pain and tenderness,
fractures and muscle weakness. However, such symptoms are rarely seen in
the elderly or, if present, are attributed to other pathology. Bone pain tends
to be diffuse and dull in nature affecting the ribcage, spine and femora,
whereas the muscle weakness, in the form of a proximal myopathy, may be
associated with wasting and hypotonia. The pain and myopathy combine
to give a waddling gait. The fractures may occur following only minimal
trauma and are particularly common in the ribs. In severe osteomalacia,
Looser's zones may form (Fig. 3.3) and fracture, particularly producing
subtrochanteric femoral neck fractures. In long-standing osteomalacia,
especially if present from childhood, bone softening may occur making
fractures rare but resulting in bony deformities such as protrusio acetabuli
or greenstick-type fractures.

Osteomalacia most likely does play a role in the aetiology of femoral
neck fractures but the extent of that role is controversial with prevalences in
various studies ranging between 2 and 25%, with the lower figures being
more generally accepted.

Rickets has most of the clinical features of osteomalacia but, in addition,
characteristic bony deformities are observed in association with growth
retardation. These include bowing of the legs, pelvic deformity, kyphosis
and scoliosis. Overproduction of osteoid in the frontal and parietal bones
produce frontal bossing, whereas overproduction of pre-osseous metaphyseal cartilage matrix produces the 'rickety rosary' deformity as well as
widening of the bones at the wrist. The clinical signs associated with
hypocalcaemia may be present, manifested by tetany and sometimes by
convulsions.

Biochemical presentation

The most common abnormality is a raised alkaline phosphatase occurring
in approximately two-thirds of adults with nutritional osteomalacia.
Serum calcium levels tend to be low normal but need correcting for
albumin levels as calcium is bound to albumin. Fasting phosphate levels

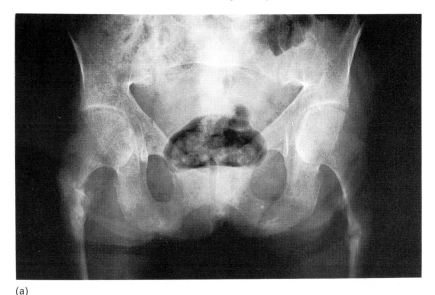

(a)

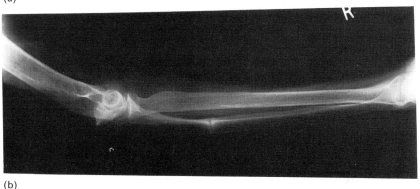

(b)

Fig. 3.3. (*a*) X-ray of pelvis showing healing Looser's zones on medical aspects of the upper femora, (*b*) X-ray showing Looser's zones in proximal ulna.

also tend to be low or low normal and thus there should be a high degree of suspicion of osteomalacia for a patient with a low normal calcium, low normal phosphate and raised alkaline phosphatase of bone origin, e.g. associated with otherwise normal liver function tests. The older the age of the patient, however, the lower the specificity of these tests become (Fig. 3.4).

25-hydroxyvitamin D (calcidiol) levels are generally unhelpful for clinical diagnosis as they are not generally available, and are expensive. In addition, studies have shown that many patients with low calcidiol levels do

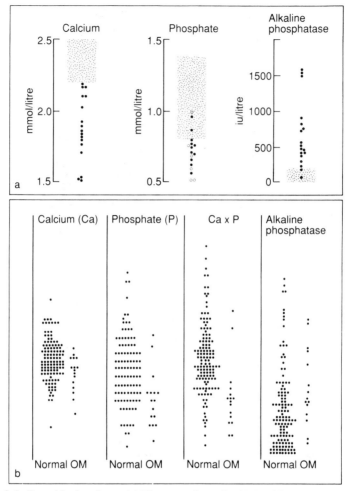

Fig. 3.4. Bone biochemistry: (*a*) Young patients (<65yr) with osteomalacia (OM) (stippled area showing normal ranges) most of whom presented with symptoms and had Looser's zones, (*b*) Elderly patients (>65yr) with and without histologically proven osteomalacia. (Reproduced by kind permission of the editors of the *British Journal of Hospital Medicine*.)

not have osteomalacia. Their use is in assessing compliance with treatment in patients with apparently unresponsive osteomalacia and for investigating the rarer causes of the disease.

1,25-dihydroxyvitamin D (calcitriol) levels are even more expensive to perform and, in addition, can be normal in the presence of histologically confirmed osteomalacia. They are helpful in the investigation of the rare causes of rickets/osteomalacia.

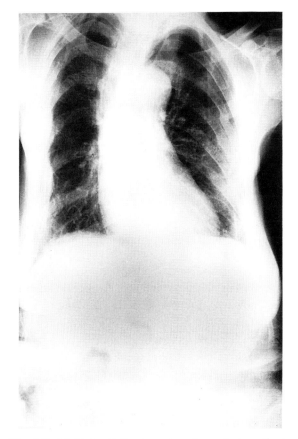

Fig. 3.5. Multiple rib fractures in osteomalacic patient.

Radiology

X-rays are generally unhelpful in identifying osteomalacic patients unless a Looser's zone (Fig. 3.3) is present. This is a translucent band of demineralised bone resulting from an unhealed cortical microfracture. However, they are only present in patients with severe longstanding disease with an estimated prevalence of 1% of affected patients. When present they are typically found in the ribs, pubic rami, scapulae and upper ends of the femora. They need to be distinguished from osteoporotic stress fractures. Perhaps the more helpful distinguishing features are the absence of a lucent band and rapid healing with callus formation in a stress fracture which, in addition, are usually solitary. Looser's zones are often multiple and symmetrical, callus is absent prior to treatment, and they are nearly always perpendicular to the periosteum.

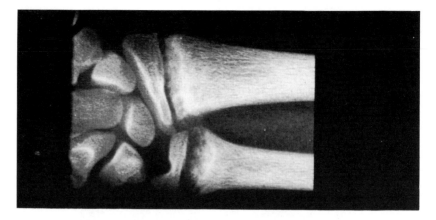

Fig. 3.6. X-ray of wrist of child with rickets.

Generalised osteopoenia with cortical thinning occurs early in the disease and may lead to multiple fractures especially in the ribs (Fig. 3.5). These changes, however, are not directly helpful in distinguishing osteomalacia from any of the other causes of osteopoenia.

In rickets, the classical radiological finding is gross widening and irregularity of the metaphyses. Cupping is best seen at the ends of the fibula or the distal ulna (Fig. 3.6).

Radionuclide scanning

A technetium-labelled diphosphonate bone scan in osteomalacic patients will show generalised tracer uptake in the axial skeleton, long bones and skull with absent kidney images. Total 24-hour retention of the isotope will also be increased. A scan is a useful investigation when used as part of a diagnostic 'work-up' for osteomalacia, but the uptake changes are not absolutely specific for osteomalacia, and isotope retention is also increased if renal failure is present. However, it may identify the presence of Looser's zones which may not have been visualised with conventional radiology as well as other suggestive signs, e.g. multiple rib fractures (Fig. 3.7) which otherwise might have been missed.

Bone biopsy

This provides the 'gold standard' for diagnosis and ideally should be performed in all suspected cases. A No. 8 Jamshidi needle (Fig. 3.8) biopsy from the anterior iliac crest will produce specimens adequate for quantitat-

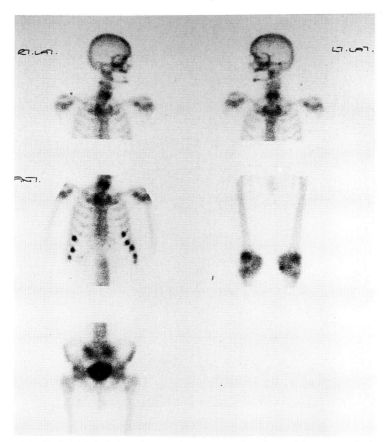

Fig. 3.7. Tc labelled diphosphonate bone scan of patient with osteomalacia and multiple rib fractures which were not visible on X-ray.

ion in most cases and, compared with a trephine biopsy, involves only minimal patient discomfort and does not require intravenous sedation. The detailed histomorphometric criteria involved in making the diagnosis are not relevant to most clinicians, but the basic requirements involve an increase in bone surface covered by osteoid in addition to an increase in the thickness of the osteoid (Fig. 3.9). In addition, evidence of decreased mineralisation activity using tetracycline labelling of the calcification front should be obtained if possible as the amount of osteoid may not reflect the extent of the mineralisation deficit. A possible tetracycline labelling regime involves giving demeclocycline 300 mg bd for 2 days followed by the bone biopsy 5 days later.

In practice, however, the facilities to cut undecalcified sections are not

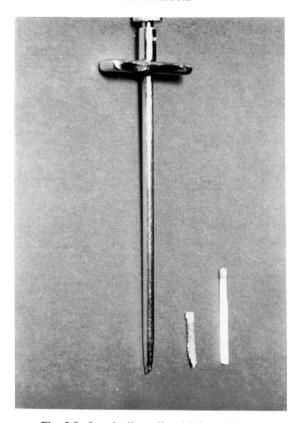

Fig. 3.8. Jamshedi needle with bone biopsy.

available in all hospitals and there is a natural reluctance to perform an invasive procedure. Similarly, although the technique for a Jamshidi biopsy is easily learnt, the average clinician may not see sufficient cases to justify use of bone biopsies if bone scanning facilities are available.

Making the diagnosis

It is essential to have a high degree of clinical suspicion for the presence of osteomalacia in any of the groups of patients summarised in Fig. 3.10. The symptoms especially in the elderly, can be non-specific and the diagnosis missed. Fig. 3.11 attempts to answer the question as to how the diagnosis of Vitamin D deficiency osteomalacia should be made. It may be necessary, if in doubt, and bone biopsy facilities are not available, to use a therapeutic trial of Vitamin D and monitor its affect on bone biochemistry. 0.5 μg of alfacalcidol daily should be used as the biochemical response appears to be

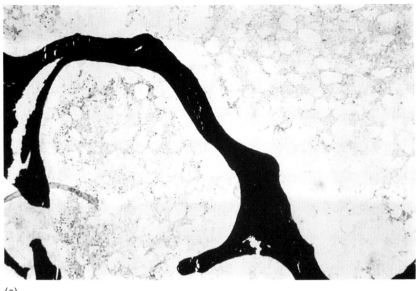

(a)

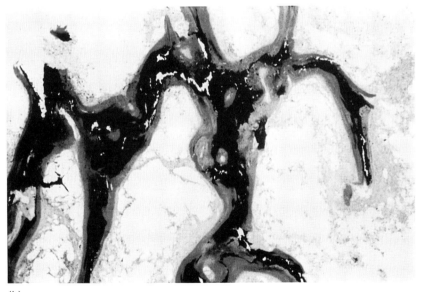

(b)

Fig. 3.9. (*a*) Normal bone (Von Kossa stain), (*b* Osteomalacic bone showing uncalcified osteoid on the bone surface (Von Kossa stain).

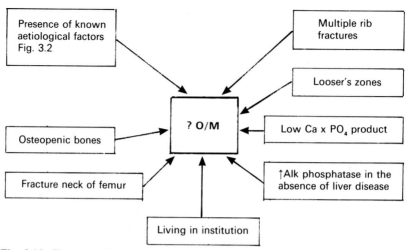

Fig. 3.10. Factors which should give rise to a clinical suspicion of osteomalacia.

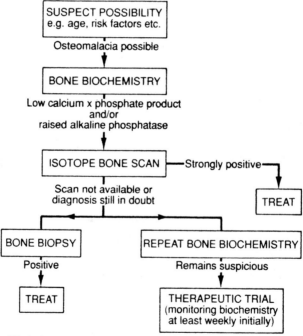

Fig. 3.11. Clinical algorithm for the management of suspected osteomalacia. (Reproduced by kind permission of the editors of the *British Journal of Hospital Medicine*.)

faster than when using calciferol. Taking blood weekly, a positive response would be a return of fasting plasma phosphate levels within a week followed by an increase in the calcium by the end of a month. After a month, there may be a small rise in alkaline phosphatase followed by a fall to a normal level in three months.

Treatment

Nutritional osteomalacia is best treated by using ergocalciferol 30 μg daily which is available in the UK in the form of calcium and Ergocalciferol tablets BPC, three daily. This will normally produce healing within three months. By using the parent compound, the risk of Vitamin D intoxication is reduced as the homeostatic safety mechanisms are not bypassed. If compliance is a problem, or if malabsorption is suspected, 600000 IU of calciferol in oil can be given IM yearly. However, absorption is unpredictable, and these patients easily become lost to follow-up on account of the infrequency of the injection.

Specific calcium supplements are generally not required apart from in severe osteomalacia where calcium uptake by bone may be so great on administration of Vitamin D that it results in severe hypocalcaemia (the hungry bone syndrome). Malabsorption syndromes can be treated with the hydroxylated metabolites which are water soluble and can be absorbed by the small intestine. There is little to choose in practice between alfacalcidol (1α-hydroxycholecalciferol) and calcitriol (1,25-dihydroxyvitamin D) but they require careful monitoring of bone biochemistry, initially weekly. Their advantage is that, if intoxication occurs, normocalcaemia returns within a few days of stopping the drug.

Hydroxylation deficiencies

Vitamin D is not metabolically active and it requires conversion initially to 25-hydroxyvitamin D in the liver and then to 1,25-dihydroxyvitamin D in the kidney. Failure of hydroxylation in either of these organs could potentially give rise to osteomalacia.

Failure of liver hydroxylation

Hepatic osteodystrophy secondary to chronic liver disease is associated with two main forms of metabolic bone disease, osteomalacia and osteoporosis, with osteoporosis being the more common disorder. Patients with chronic cholestatic liver disease, e.g. primary biliary cirrhosis are particularly prone to develop osteomalacia, but the consensus is that failure of hepatic hydroxylation is not the major aetiological factor, as 25-hydroxylation in the liver has been shown to remain adequate even in the presence of severe hepatic dysfunction. Such patients are often chronically ill and their osteomalacia is probably predominantly caused by poor sunlight exposure and dietary deprivation. This theory is supported by the fact that the majority of studies documenting convincing hepatic osteomalacia are confined to countries where privational osteomalacia is seen. In contrast, few cases have been reported in the USA where there is widespread Vitamin D supplementation of foodstuffs. It is worth noting that it has been demonstrated that the presence of jaundice does not affect the cutaneous synthesis of cholecalciferol. Other probable aetiological factors include the consequences of malabsorption of Vitamin D due to bile acid deficiency, often exacerbated by the use of bile acid binding resins such as choles-tyramine, used to control pruritus. In alcoholic liver disease, impaired 25-hydroxylation has been described, although nutritional deficiency and impairment of Vitamin D absorption are probably the major aetiological factors.

'**Anti-convulsant osteomalacia**,' found in some patients on long-term anti-convulsant therapy, has been attributed to increased turnover of 25 hydroxy vitamin D secondary to the induction of hepatic microsomal enzymes. This increases the percentage (normally 70%) of Vitamin D converted to more water soluble metabolites and excreted in the bile. However, 25-hydroxy vitamin D levels are often normal in these patients and, whereas phenobarbitone has been shown to enhance Vitamin D catabolism, phenytoin, which is more often associated with osteomalacia, does not appear to do so. Phenytoin may, however, contribute to lowering serum calcium levels by a direct effect on intestinal calcium absorption, and it has been postulated that a combination of enzyme inducing agents is required to convert a borderline Vitamin D depletion state into frank deficiency. Thus lack of sunlight exposure and poor diet are the most likely aetiological factors in patients with osteomalacia on anticonvulsants. Treatment with calciferol in adequate doses is effective.

Failure of renal hydroxylation

Failure to hydroxylate 25-hydroxy vitamin D by a 1α-hydroxylase in the kidney is most commonly the result of chronic renal failure (see Chapter 6). Even in the healthy elderly, 1,25-dihydroxy vitamin D levels are lower than in the young which may be a further possible contributory factor for the increased prevalence of osteomalacia in the elderly.

There is also a very rare congenital deficiency of 1α hydroxylase giving rise to a disease known as *Vitamin D dependency rickets Type I*. It is an autosomal recessive disorder usually presenting in the first year of life although cases have been described presenting in early adulthood. Clinically, it presents with the features of Vitamin D deficiency rickets, e.g. hypotonia, myopathy, convulsions and growth retardation. Biochemically, there is hypocalcaemia, a raised alkaline phosphatase, generalised aminoaciduria and there may be hypophosphataemia. Serum 25-hydroxy vitamin D levels are, however, normal (they would be low in Vitamin D deficiency) but 1,25-hydroxy vitamin D levels are low. It responds to treatment with physiological doses of calcitriol (0.5 μg–2 μg/day). Calcium supplementation is often required initially to correct the hypocalcaemia.

End organ resistance

Vitamin D dependency rickets Type II is a very rare form of end organ resistance osteomalacia probably caused by faulty binding to tissue receptors. It has an autosomal recessive inheritance, and parental consanguinity appears to be an important factor. It presents as rickets in the first year of life with most of the biochemical characteristics of the Type I disorder. In contrast, however, 1,25 Vitamin D levels are markedly elevated (up to × 1000 normal values). In addition, about half the cases often have and scalp alopecia, which usually is indicative of a more severe form of the disease with poor response to treatment. The condition sometimes responds to huge doses of calcitriol (20–60 μg/day) with calcium supplementation. In some cases, spontaneous recovery has been reported.

Hypophosphataemic states

Phosphate is required for normal bone mineralisation, and many conditions giving rise to phosphate depletion may give rise to osteomalacia. These conditions are characterised by significant hypophosphataemia with normal serum calcium levels with alkaline phosphatase levels tending to be higher in children who present with rickets than in adults.

X-linked hypophosphataemic rickets (familial vitamin D resistant rickets is generally an X-linked dominant disorder characterised by hypophosphataemia, ligamental calcification, osteosclerosis, impaired bone mineralisatioin and retarded growth usually presenting in early infancy. Although all affected exhibit hypophosphataemia, the conditions varies in the severity of the bone disease with males being more severely affected than females. The condition occasionally presents for the first time in adult life. The basic defect consists of a renal phosphate leak and defective 1,25 Vitamin D production. Biochemically the untreated patient will have hypophosphataemia, normocalcaemia and a raised alkaline phosphatase with elevated urinary phosphate levels. Normally, hypophosphataemia would stimulate 1,25 hydroxy vitamin D production but 1,25 hydroxy vitamin D levels have been found to be either normal or low normal suggesting an additional abnormality of defective 1,25-hydroxy Vitamin D production. Clinically, although affected children have the skeletal deformities of rickets, they do not have the myopathy, convulsions or tetany associated withy Vitamin D deficiency rickets. In adults, the ligamentous ossification can give rise to severe disability with pain and limitation of movement of affected sites. The osteosclerosis may mimic the radiological appearance of osteopetrosis or renal osteodystrophy. Treatment consists of phosphate supplements in divided doses throughout the day in order to maintain normal serum phosphate levels (30–130 mmol/day and calcitriol 1–2 µg/day).

Tumour-induced osteomalacia generally occurs between the ages of 20 and 50 y and present as osteomalacia with phosphaturia with no previous history of childhood rickets, growth retardation or family involvement (distinguishing it from a heriditary hypophosphataemia). It is caused by usually benign, often vascular, tumours of predominantly mesenchymal origin, e.g. haemangiomas, giant cell tumours secreting an, as yet, unidentified phosphaturic factor. It does not appear to be a PTH analogue as, unlike PTH, it inhibits synthesis of 1,25-hydroxyvitamin D as well as appearing to have little effect on calcium transport. The tumours may be undetectable and be located within otherwise normal bones. Clinically patients present with bone pain, myopathy and fractures often through Looser's zones with generalised osteopoenia. Serum phosphate levels are characteristically very low, serum calcium is normal and alkaline phosphatase levels raised. Cure is achieved by recognising and resecting the tumour. If this cannot be achieved, treatment with phosphate supplements and calcitriol (1–2 µg/day) is successful.

Fanconi syndrome may be idiopathic or associated with inborn errors of metabolism (e.g. Wilson's Disease, cystinosis) or acquired conditions (e.g. heavy metal poisoning, drug-related or paraproteinaemias). Decreased tubular reabsorption of phosphate is amongst the manifestations of proximal renal tubular dysfunction. In addition the accompanying acidosis may itself give rise to rickets/osteomalacia, possibly through inhibition of 1,25-hydroxy vitamin D synthesis or by dissolution of bone mineral from hydroxyapatite crystals which act as a buffer for excess acid. The X-ray findings are classically those of rickets/osteomalacia associated with nephrocalcinosis. Treatment of the rickets/osteomalacia is with calcitriol and phosphate supplements, although the underlying disease process is usually the predominant clinical problem.

Bone poisons

Impaired mineralisation can be caused by several drugs.

(i) Sodium editronate when used in high doses for the treatment of Paget's disease may result in poor mineralisation but is rare with doses of 5 mg/kg/day if used for a maximum of six months. Newer bisphosphonates may be free of this side-effect but are not licensed yet for Paget's disease.

(ii) Sodium fluoride given in large doses for the treatment of osteoporosis may induce osteomalacia. The osteomalacic component of fluorosis is only rarely symptomatic, however, although it may contribute to the increased vertebral fracture rate seen in the first year of fluoride treatment.

(iii) Aluminium, obtained from the dialysis fluid or phosphate binders (e.g. aluminium hydroxide) in patients in chronic renal failure, is a potent inhibitor of mineralisation as well as matrix synthesis by the osteoblasts. This gives rise histologically to 'aplastic' or low-turnover osteomalacia with minimal osteoid formation and reduced bone turnover. Aluminium is found to accumulate at the mineralisation front preventing calcium deposition and may inhibit PTH production by accumulating in parathyroid tissue. It may be this latter effect which allows the production of a histologically predominantly 'pure' osteomalacia without the changes of osteitis fibrosa in chronic renal failure.

Miscellaneous

Osteomalacia associated with chronic metabolic acidosis and long term dialysis is described elsewhere (under Fanconi syndrome and Renal Bone Disease, respectively).

Osteomalacia has been reported in patients receiving **Chronic parenteral nutrition** presents clinically with severe bone pain and histologically with an 'aplastic' picture. Its aetiology is uncertain.

Hypophosphatasia is an autosomal recessive disorder which presents in the neonatal period or early infancy with rickets. It is discussed in greater detail in Chapter 2.

82 *Osteomalacia*

Further reading

Campbell, G.A. (1990). Osteomalacia–diagnosis and management. *British Journal of Hospital Medicine*, **44**, 332–8.

Parfitt, A.M. (1990). Osteomalacia and related disorders. In *Metabolic Bone Disease and Clinically Related Disorders*. 2nd edn. eds. Avioli, L.V. & Krane, S.M. W.B. Saunders Company, pp. 329–396.

Anast, C.N., Carpenter, T.O. & Key, L.L. (1990). Metabolic bone disorders in children. In *Metabolic Bone Disease and Clinically Related Disorders*. 2nd edn. eds. Avioli, L.V. & Krane, S.M. W.B. Saunders Company, pp. 329–396.

4

Paget's disease

Introduction and epidemiology

On 14 November 1876, Sir James Paget, a surgeon of St Bartholomew's Hospital, delivered the first comprehensive account of *osteitis deformans*, the name which is still curiously preferred by *Index Medicus*, to the Medical and Chirurgical Society of London. Paget's disease is a chronic non-inflammatory disorder characterised by accelerated resorption and production of bone, resulting in deformity and fragility and, in Paget's own phrase, by 'change of size, shape and direction'.

The disease rarely presents before the age of 40. The rare condition, idiopathic hyperphosphatasia (sometimes called juvenile Paget's) is characterised by bone deformity in childhood and a likely recessive inheritance and is probably unrelated to adult Paget's disease. Autopsy studies suggest that its prevalence approximately doubles with each decade after the age of 50 and may affect more than 10% of our population over the age of 95. The most comprehensive surveys were based on limited skeletal surveys of radiographs on hospital inpatients and one might very reasonably conclude that these results underestimate the prevalence of Paget's disease. William Barker conducted a survey of British patients of 55 years and over in 31 towns and concluded that 4–5% had Paget's disease with a focus in Lancashire of 7–8% (Fig. 4.1). There are likely to be almost a million people in Britain with Paget's disease.

About 10–30% of patients have a single Pagetic lesion (monostotic disease) and the rest polyostotic disease. A slight male preponderance has usually been accepted with a male:female ratio of about 3:2 but increasingly referral centres are documenting an approximately equal incidence in both sexes. This may reflect the relative longevity of women. There have been many reports of Paget's disease in several members of the same family whether children, siblings or parents, but only five pairs of identical twins with the disease have been documented. The present author has seen three

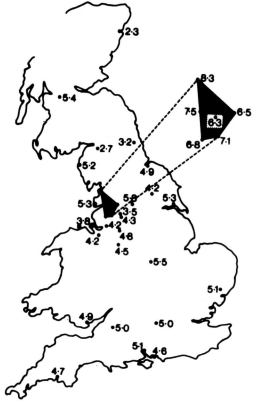

Fig. 4.1. The prevalence of (%) of Paget's disease in hospital patients over 55 years. (By permission of Professor William Barker of Southampton and the *British Medical Journal* (1980) **280**, 1105–7.)

brothers from Cornwall who all developed Paget's disease below the age of 40, and who all developed osteosarcomas. Genetic factors do seem to play a part in at least some cases of this disease. One study suggested that parents and siblings of affected patients had a 10-fold greater chance of having Paget's disease when compared with the parents and siblings of the normal spouse. HLA A9 and B15 are increased in patients when compared with a control population in Sheffield. The most striking epidemiological feature of Paget's disease is its preponderance in Britain, North America, Australia and New Zealand, and its relative rarity in Eire, Scandinavia, Asia and in non-white races. This would imply that Paget's is a genetically determined disorder which has been disseminated by the migration of populations and perhaps originated many generations ago in Britain. Pagetic skeletons have been identified from the 10th century AD.

Kanis argues that the incidence of Paget's disease may now be

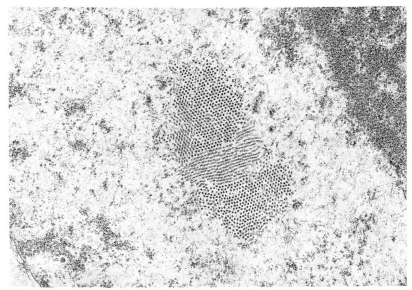

Fig. 4.2. Viral-like inclusion bodies in a Pagetic osteoclast nucleus by electron microscopy. (By permission of Professor Andre Rebel of Angers, France.)

decreasing. Its declining report on death certificates is unreliable, but there is a decreasing number of deaths attributed to adult osteosarcomas which may be a marker for the underlying incidence of Paget's disease as most cases in adult life arise from Pagetic bone.

Pathogenesis

Histopathology

Paget's disease is characterised by the increased metabolic activity of bone. Bone remodelling usually occurs on less than 10% of the bone surface but, in Pagetic bone, up to 100% of the bone surface can be involved in resorption or new bone formation. This is caused by increased 'activation frequency' of the bone remodelling units (BMU) so that the quiescent periods which normal bone experience are much shorter.

The striking histological feature of the disease is the increased number and size of osteoclasts which mediate bone resorption. Osteoclasts may be increased up to 100-fold and the size and number of their nuclei are also inflated. An osteoclast may contain up to 100 nuclei. Electron microscopy of osteoclast nuclei demonstrates virus-like inclusions [Fig. 4.2].

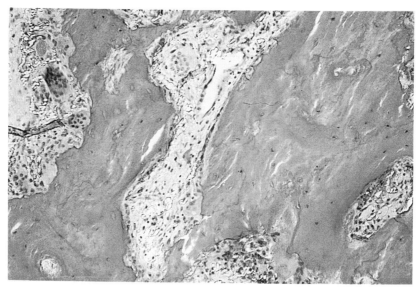

Fig. 4.3. A photomicrograph of Pagetic bone. (By permission of Oxford University Press; chapter by A.J. Crisp, *Oxford Textbook of Rheumatology*.)

Resorption by the large 'angry' osteoclasts of Pagetic bone is followed by active bone formation as these processes, even in pathological bone remodelling, are virtually always closely linked. The common exception to this principle is myeloma in which the osteoblastic response may be muted or absent. Pagetic osteoblasts are increased in size and number but do not contain virus-like inclusions. They are often pleomorphic. Osteoblasts in Paget's disease characteristically make woven bone which is not usually present in the adult except during fracture repair and in other high turnover states such as hyperparathyroidism or renal osteodystrophy. This disrupts the normal lamellar structure of the matrix collagen with increased intraosseous fibrosis, hyper-vascularity and enlarged haversian canals. This disordered bone has a lower and more variable mineral content and is consequently weaker. Pagetic bone consists of a variable mixture of immature ('woven') bone and irregular mature lamellar bone (without haversian systems) separated by deeply staining cement lines in the characteristic mosaic pattern of the disease (Fig. 4.3).

Aetiology

The intriguing clues that genetic factors may play a major part in the aetiology of Paget's disease have been discussed above. However, there is much to commend the view that a slow virus infection of bone cells is also a *sine qua non.* The viral inclusions virtually always identified in some osteoclast nuclei by electron microscopy have a consistent appearance. They comprise micro-cylinders found as loose filaments or in a paracrystal-line arrangement with the size and periodicity characteristic of para-myxoviral nucleocapsids. These can also occur in the cytoplasm. An early morphological link was made with the inclusions found in the brain cells of patients with subacute sclerosing panencephalitis, a known sequela of measles. Closely related paramyxoviruses include respiratory syncytial virus [RSV] and canine distemper virus, and each virus has been proposed as the infectious trigger for Paget's disease in individuals genetically predisposed.

A causal link between the viral inclusions and Paget's disease has not been established yet. Immunohistochemical studies have provided further tantalising evidence. Polyclonal antibodies reveal paramyxovirus antigen in Pagetic osteoclasts compatible with measles and RSV, and studies with monoclonal antibodies implicate measles, simian virus and human parain-fluenza. *In situ* hybridisation with DNA probes specific for measles nucleocapsid protein detects measles sequences in osteoclasts but probes also hybridise with osteoblasts, fibroblasts and lymphocytes which raise doubts about specificity.

David Anderson's group in Manchester are actively pursuing the canine distemper virus (CDV) as the causative virus. Early epidemiological studies attempted to link dog ownership in early life with the later development of Paget's disease and recently probes have detected the RNA of the CDV nucleocapsid in over half of Pagetic bone biopsies.

There are many factors arguing against this slow virus hypothesis. There is little serological evidence for these virus infections when sera are examined from Pagetic patients and controls. Attempts to recover virus from Pagetic cells or from Pagetic osteosarcomata have met with abject failure as have attempts to passage the disease to uninfected cell cultures and animals. This is not necessarily damning evidence as the high mutation rate of viral RNA is notorious. The viral inclusion may just represent a marker of past active infection. However, the immune modulator, inosiplex, has some activity against subacute sclerosing panencephalitis of measles but has no effect in Paget's disease.

If one accepts the viral hypothesis, it is worth considering Kahn's suggestion that the target cell for viral infection may not be the osteoclast, to which has been directed most attention, but the osteoblast. The structure of the osteoblast is more deranged in Paget's disease than in other high-turnover states such as renal osteodystrophy. Common progenitor cells give rise to osteoclasts, granulocytes and monocytes and distribute their progeny widely throughout the circulation. One might then expect that new bone involvement would be 'metastatic' in each patient which is incorrect. Osteoblasts, which are modified fibroblasts, proliferate locally, and this would be more compatible with the pattern of bone involvement in Paget's disease.

Relatively little is known about the molecular basis of Paget's disease. Growth factors and cytokines, such as interleukin 6, are bound to be implicated in the anarchic processes of the disease which are characterised by bone destruction without respect for the existing architecture and neovascularisation. Non-transforming and transforming growth factors (known to be secreted by some osteosarcoma cells) are likely participants in this disease which some consider to be a benign tumour of bone.

Clinical features

Many patients with Paget's disease are unaware of it. If one accepts the viral aetiology, it is likely that infection occurs in early life, and many years pass before bone lesions are detectable. The diagnosis is often made incidentally during radiological or biochemical investigation of other systems. The Pagetic vertebra seen on a plain abdominal radiograph or a raised serum alkaline phosphatase are very common presenting features. Although long-term prospective studies of outcome in asymptomatic patients with Paget's disease have not been made, perhaps only 10–20% of patients will eventually develop clinical symptoms or signs clearly attributable to the disease.

Apart from fracture the onset of symptoms is usually insidious and about 30% of patients have had symptoms at presentation for more than 10 years. A minority have had symptoms for 30 years or more and 7% have symptoms which were present before the age of 40, which argues that the possible diagnosis of Paget's disease should not be ignored in younger patients.

The clinical features of Paget's disease are outlined in Table 4.1. The presenting features of the disease in one large series are presented in Table 4.2, and the skeletal distribution of lesions in Table 4.3.

Pain

Bone pain

Pain is the most common presenting symptom and can arise from any affected bone. It is often difficult to be certain whether pain is arising from

Table. 4.1. *Clinical features of Paget's disease*

Pain	• Pagetic • adjacent joint (usually secondary osteoarthritis with or without pyrophosphate arthropathy)
Bone expansion and deformity	
Fractures	• long bones (complete or incomplete 'fissure fractures') • crush fractures of vertebral bodies
Heat	
Neurological syndromes	• deafness (most common) • headache • tinnitus • vertigo • spinal cord and root compression • brainstem/cerebellar compression • visual impairment • other cranial nerve involvement
Malignant osteosarcoma and benign giant cell tumour	
Immobilisation hypercalcaemia and hypercalciuria	• renal stone formation • primary hyperparathyroidism more common than chance?
High output cardiac failure	
Hyperuricaemia and gout Angioid streaks of retina	• controversial

Table. 4.2. *The presenting features of Paget's disease in a series of 197 Sheffield patients (after Kanis)*

	%
Pain	86
Deformity	17
Asymptomatic	12
Neurological	17
• cranial nerve	11
• spinal cord or root	5
• peripheral nerve	1
Fracture	11
Other	3
Tumour	1

Table. 4.3. *Distribution of Paget's disease in the skeleton*

	%
Pelvis	72–76
Lumbar spine	33–58
Thoracic spine	24–45
Femur	25–55
Sacrum	29–44
Skull	28–42
Tibia	22–35
Radius	16
Feet	10
Hands	9
Ribs	3

bone itself or from the adjacent joint. It is often multifactorial. Typically, the bone pain of Paget's disease is constant, deep and boring, sometimes worse at night and at rest. The cause of pain is not well understood but is likely to be related to increased bone and periosteal blood flow in metabolically active bone increasing intraosseous pressure and stimulating bone pain fibres in canaliculi.

Thermographic studies of the tibia suggest that pain is related to temperature which reflects both skin and bone blood flow. It is known that the drilling of affected bone may reduce pain, and studies with rapidly acting drugs, such as mithramycin (plicamycin) suggest a correlation between pain relief and the reduction of bone blood flow as indicated by thermography.

Adjacent joint pain

A major cause of pain is adjacent joint disease. Bone deformity commonly alters force transmission through the adjacent joint causing premature loss of articular cartilage and secondary osteoarthritis especially at hip and knee. Patients can also develop osteoarthritis in an unaffected knee as a result of favouring the contralateral, non-Pagetic knee. Metabolically active, hyperaemic, subchondral bone may also be toxic to articular cartilage. Osteoarthritic pain is usually associated with exercise and relieved by rest and sleep but it is often very difficult to dissociate bone pain from joint pain. It is sometimes useful to inject lignocaine into the joint. If the pain is unaffected then a bone origin for the pain may be inferred.

Protrusio acetabuli occurs in about one-quarter of hip joints involved by Paget's disease presumably because of bone softening. There is no evidence that the natural history of the osteoarthritis can be affected by medical treatment of the Pagetic bone. Sir James Paget and others since claimed that hyperuricaemia and gout are increased in these patients, but there is little recent evidence to support this association. An increased incidence of chondrocalcinosis and pyrophosphate arthropathy (with acute pseudogout) has also been claimed but there is little to support this link. The commonest cause of chondrocalcinosis is osteoarthritis itself which is therefore a confusing variable.

Back pain in patients with Paget's disease is often difficult to analyse. Pain may arise from vertebral body expansion caused by bone involvement, and also from the frank crush fracture or microfracture of the body caused by bone weakness. Independent or associated degenerative spondylosis with osteoarthritic expansion of facet joints and osteophytes is often also present and, if particularly exuberant, may progress to ankylosing hyperostosis (Forestier's disease). These processes can all cause spinal cord or nerve root involvement and comprehensive examination and investigation will be necessary to determine appropriate management.

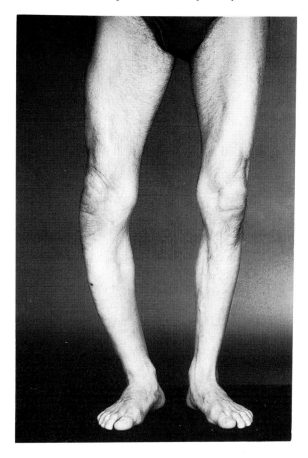

Fig. 4.4. A patient with Paget's disease showing the bowing and external rotation of the right femur. He complained of osteoarthritic pain in right knee and ankle and burning pain in the lower leg. Paget's disease was present in the right femur and tibia. (By permission of Oxford University Press: chapter by A.J. Crisp, *Oxford Textbook of Rheumatology*.)

Bone expansion and deformity

Bone enlargement and deformity is usually the most obvious and reliable physical sign of Paget's disease. It is the cause of much neurological involvement and of long bone abnormalities. The most frequent deformity of long bones is bowing which is characteristically lateral in the femur and anterior in the tibia (Fig. 4.4). This can cause inequality of leg length

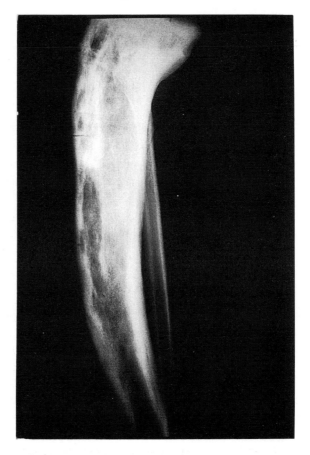

Fig. 4.5. The lateral radiograph of a Pagetic right tibia with fissure fractures. (By permission of Dr David Moore of Sheffield.)

leading to lumbar scoliosis and accelerated degenerative lumbar spondylosis. Adaptation to slow, insidious deformity may cause remarkably few symptoms, but gross bowing may allow only a 'scissor gait' which makes walking virtually impossible.

The skin overlying bowed Pagetic bone often seems to be compromised in spite of increased vascular nutrition, and can ulcerate or heal poorly after minor injury.

Skull deformities are variable and characteristic. Anterior bossing of the skull caused by calvarial thickening is common. Expansion of the upper or lower jaw can cause dental malocclusion and probably the most unacceptable 'cosmetic' abnormalities.

Fractures

In one series of 180 patients, 15% suffered pathological fractures in abnormal bone. There are three common types: fissure fractures, fractures of long bones and vertebral body compression fractures.

Fissure fractures

These are common and involve long bones, especially femur, tibia and humerus (Fig. 4.5). They can also occur in the pelvis, but their presence at that site should stimulate investigation for vitamin D deficiency ('Looser's zones'). Fissure fractures may be asymptomatic or painful. When pain develops at the site of a known fissure fracture, this may herald complete fracture, and dynamic bracing at this site may be indicated. Healing or partial healing of fissure fractures is observed, but there is no convincing evidence that specific medical treatment affects this.

Complete fractures

These are most common in femur, tibia and forearm and can, to some extent, be predicted by radiographic appearances. Trauma is often trivial. In Paget's disease, subtrochanteric and femoral shaft fractures are more common than femoral neck fractures which are more characteristic of osteoporosis. Unlike fractures of normal bones, complete fractures through Pagetic long bones are usually transverse rather than spiral. Complete fracture through Pagetic bone should always trigger the thought of underlying sarcoma especially in the humerus.

Most completed fractures heal well with closed or surgical reduction but the incidence of non-union may be up to 40%. This may argue that the presence of fissure fractures which might be expected to lead to complete fractures should be treated more aggressively.

Other fractures

Vertebral body compression fractures are common. The presence of osteolysis may be confused with osteoporosis and the clinical consequences: pain, kyphosis and loss of height are similar.

Heat

Palpation of affected bones near to skin surfaces often reveals temperature asymmetry. Bone tenderness is unusual. Auscultation of the tibia or skull

Table. 4.4. *The mechanisms and signs of neurological involvement in Paget's disease*

Skull	
Deformity of skull base (platybasia)	Acute brainstem compression
	Cranial nerve syndromes
	Upper motor neurone signs
	Raised intracranial pressure
	Vascular compression
Narrowing of cranial nerve foramina	I, II, V, VII, VIII lower motor neurone lesions
Hyperaemia of skull vault	'Steal' syndromes, confusion, ataxia, dementia
Vertebrae	
Bone entrapment of spinal cord or nerve roots and vascular 'steal'	Quadriparesis
	Paraparesis
	Cauda equina syndrome
	Root pain

can sometimes reveal bruits. Temperature may be correlated with both metabolic activity of bone and with bone pain.

Neurological syndromes

These are summarised in Table 4.4.

Platybasia and cranial nerve syndromes

Platybasia is invagination of the skull base caused by bone softening and can cause pressure of the odontoid peg on the brainstem. This can precipitate ataxia, weakness with long tract compression and respiratory insufficiency, vertebrobasilar insufficiency and cerebellar syndromes. Vague neurological syndromes – headache, confusion and ataxia – are common in the elderly and occur in Paget's disease. They can perhaps be linked with vascular steal syndromes.

Deafness

This occurs in up to half the patients with skull involvement. A Menière's-like syndrome of headache, vertigo, tinnitus, nausea and vomiting can rarely occur. The deafness is sensorineural, conductive or mixed. Bony encroachment on the internal auditory canal by the petrous temporal bone can occur and the cochlea can also be compressed. Subtle toxic effects on the inner ear mediated by hypervascularity are also likely. Conductive hearing loss may also result from involvement of the ossicles of the middle ear, resulting in ankylosis and rigidity of the foot plate of the stapes.

Other cranial nerve lesions

Narrowing of the optic foramen may produce papilloedema and optic atrophy but blindness, which Paget himself first described, is very rare. Although the angioid streaks which are seen in Bruch's membrane of the retina in many patients with Paget's disease are not a cranial nerve lesion, they are worth mentioning here. These streaks can suggest that there is a generalised connective tissue disorder in Paget's disease.

Other cranial nerve lesions have been rarely described causing anosmia, trigeminal neuralgia, facial palsy or bulbar palsy with dysphagia.

Spinal disease

This has been briefly considered above. Spinal cord compression is quite rare when one considers the frequency of vertebral Paget's disease. Bone encroachment may play a part but vascular steal syndromes are now considered to be more important in the episode of acute neurological cord dysfunction as they may often respond to medical treatment. In some patients, no anatomical obstruction has been found by myelography or scanning arguing for a more subtle, vascular mechanism.

Anatomical cord compression is most likely to occur in the thoracic spine where the vertebral canal is narrowest and often only one thoracic vertebra is involved. Sometimes, recurrent surgical decompressive laminectomy is required. The present author has a patient who has undergone three cervical operations to decompress her spinal cord in spite of aggressive medical therapy. Cord involvement is typically insidious rather than acute.

Cardiovascular involvement

When more than one-third of the skeleton is involved by Paget's disease, high output cardiac failure has been rarely reported. The prevalence of aortic valve calcification has been claimed to be increased fourfold in patients with Paget's disease.

Neoplastic complications

Many cases of osteosarcoma in adults arise from Pagetic bone, but conversely osteosarcoma is a very rare complication of Paget's disease occurring in about 0.1% of affected patients. Almost all patients with skull osteosarcoma have the disease. Paget's probably carries a 30-fold increase in risk for osteosarcoma. The pelvis and femur are common sites followed by the humerus, face and skull. Fibrosarcoma, chondrosarcoma and reticulosarcoma are much rarer developments.

Not all tumours arising from Paget's bone are malignant. Benign giant cell tumours which may be indistinguishable from reparative granulomas are also well described. They are most often found in the skull and face and sometimes are only cured by radical excision of the tumour. Some giant cell tumours respond to radiotherapy and corticosteroids. One interesting American series of patients with giant cell tumours arising from Pagetic bone traced a common origin for some of the patients from Avellino in Italy. A similar patient from Avellino has been recently reported from Britain.

The diagnosis of maligant osteosarcoma is worth considering in a patient who develops intense pain in an affected bone with a progressive lytic lesion and a rising alkaline phosphatase against a background of stable symptoms. Radiographs, as well as showing active bone lysis, may reveal a soft tissue tumour which can be confirmed by scanning (Fig. 4.6). Open or needle biopsy will prove the diagnosis. Pagetic osteosarcomas carry a poor prognosis with only 10% 5-year survival figures. One reason for the usually rapid deterioration of these patients is the early metastatic spread from highly vascular sites.

Immobilisation, hypercalcaemia and hypercalciuria

The serum calcium concentration is usually normal but during immobilisation for an unrelated illness, fracture or elective orthopaedic surgery, hypercalciuria and, less commonly, hypercalcaemia, can occur. Bone formation is inhibited but resorption continues unchecked. Rarely, both abnormalities can occur without immobilisation, but this can often be traced to underlying primary hyperparathyroidism which may occur more frequently than one would expect by chance association.

Hypercalciuria clearly predisposes to renal stone formation but it has been claimed that Paget's disease may be associated with a variety of examples of extraskeletal calcification: aortic valve and vascular calcification, chondrocalcinosis, salivary stones and cutaneous calcification. These associations remain unproven.

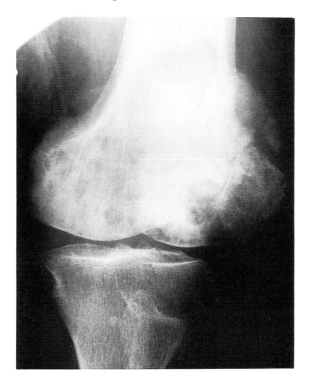

Fig. 4.6. Radiograph of an osteosarcoma with a soft tissue mass arising from a Pagetic distal femur. (By permission of Dr David Moore of Sheffield.)

Investigations and assessment

The discovery of Paget's disease in a patient, whether this has been accidental in an asymptomatic patient or directed by a presenting symptom or sign, should lead on to an adequate assessment of the patient in 'routine' clinical practice. It is highly desirable to know the anatomical extent of the disease so that later clinical events can be interpreted correctly and also the biochemical activity of the disease. A minimum programme of investigation should therefore comprise:

- full blood count
- erythrocyte sedimentation rate [ESR]
- urea and electrolytes
- liver function tests
- serum calcium, phosphate and alkaline phosphatase
- 24-hour urine hydroxyproline/creatinine ratio (if available)

- isotope bone scan, to locate the number and extent of Pagetic bone lesions
- plain radiographs of all affected sites localised by isotope bone scan to document lytic areas, fissure fractures and osteosarcomas and the extent of osteoarthritis
- specific investigations, e.g. audiometry, for patients with skull involvement

This baseline information will then allow rational treatment decisions to be made. These investigational techniques will now be considered in more detail.

Biochemical investigation

Serum calcium, parathyroid hormone (PTH) and calcitonin

In spite of the skeletal chaos induced by widespread Paget's disease, serum calcium typically remains within the normal range, and this is a tribute to the sensitive metabolic mechanisms which exist to maintain normocalcaemia. Hypercalcaemia is very rare and usually only occurs in the immobilised patient when bone formation is inhibited in the presence of continuing reabsorption. Resorption is also inhibited in the normal person but in Paget's disease this process seems more autonomous.

Raised serum concentrations of PTH (employing some assays) have been found in up to a quarter of patients with extensive Paget's disease, but normocalcaemia is usually maintained. Newer radioimmunoassays measuring intact PTH (as opposed to region specific assays) usually document normal values but a higher incidence of hyperparathyroidism in patients with Paget's disease than expected has been claimed.

Serum concentrations of calcitonin are normal in Paget's disease and there is no evidence for deficiency. The daily secretion rate of calcitonin in physiological states is about 13 units or less compared with therapeutic doses of 50 units or more.

Serum alkaline phosphatase

This osteoblastic enzyme, a measure of new bone formation and not resorption, is the most useful and widely available marker and may be elevated by as much as 30 times above the upper limit of the reference range. The function of this enzyme remains unclear but one substrate is inorganic pyrophosphate, a known inhibitor of calcification, and alkaline phosphatase seems to be a key enzyme in mineralisation processes. In most clinical biochemistry laboratories, total alkaline phosphatase is measured; about half is bone derived and half derived from liver with a small component from intestine and a larger component from placenta during pregnancy. Analysis of isoenzymes of alkaline phosphatase or measurement of alternative liver enzymes (e.g. gamma glutamyl transpeptidase, 5-nucleotidase) help to exclude a significant hepatic contribution to the total alkaline phosphatase.

The turnover of bone alkaline phosphatase is rapid with a half-life of 1–2 days which makes serum measurements an effective reflection of osteoblast activity. There is little diurnal variation but the within-patient coefficient of variation is about 10%. There is a significant correlation between alkaline phosphatase and the extent of skeletal involvement by Paget's disease and with urine hydroxyproline excretion. Occasionally, alkaline phosphatase is normal with limited Paget's disease, but one should not be deterred by a normal result from treating a painful Pagetic lesion.

Urine hydroxyproline

Increased osteoclastic bone resorption parallels increased bone formation and may be assessed by assay of urine hydroxyproline excretion, a breakdown product of collagen. Most hydroxyproline of endogenous origin that is excreted in urine comes from bone and skin but probably only 20% of total hydroxyproline measured in urine derives from newly resorbed bone. These measurements are associated with a number of other difficulties. It is a laborious technique and is less widely available than alkaline phosphatase. Ideally, the patient should have followed a gelatin (denatured-collagen)-free diet for 48 hours before the urine collection to exclude a dietary contribution but this is often impractical. The variable compliance of patients in excluding meat, jelly, icecream and gravy from their diets somewhat impairs the reliability of this test. The urine hydroxyproline/creatinine ratio may also be determined on a fasting overnight spot urine collection which makes this a more practical exercise.

Urine pyridinoline collagen cross-links

The recent development of assays to measure the excretion of bone specific collagen cross-links offers the prospect of accurate measurement of current osteoclastic bone resorption. Unlike hydroxyproline, these are not metabolised and measurements are not confounded by new synthesis of the measured metabolite. It is widely considered that these assays will rapidly replace urine hydroxyproline as a useful osteoclastic function test.

Serum osteocalcin

This is also known as bone gamma-carboxyglutamic acid containing protein (BGP) and is a vitamin K-dependent protein with a high affinity for hydroxyapatite. It is the main non-collagenous protein in bone and is produced specifically by osteoblasts. It showed promise as a specific marker for bone formation, but only half the patients with Paget's disease with raised alkaline phosphatase also have raised osteocalcin concentrations. Values can be increased by treatment via interactions between parathyroid hormone and 1,25 dihydroxyvitamin D. Osteocalcin is unlikely to offer any advantages over conventional indices of disease activity in Paget's disease.

Serum acid phosphatase

Osteoclasts are rich in acid phosphatase, and some patients with Paget's disease have raised levels. Occasionally, metastatic carcinoma of the prostate is incorrectly diagnosed in the presence of sclerotic vertebrae and elevated acid phosphatase. The two conditions may co-exist by chance and cause diagnostic difficulty. Acid phosphatase is not a helpful index of osteoclast activity.

Alpha 2 HS-glycoprotein

This liver derived protein is taken up by active bone, and concentrations tend to be lower than normal in active Paget's disease. The sensitivity and specificity of this measurement are too low for this test to be reliable in Paget's disease.

Uric acid

The increased nucleic acid turnover in Paget's disease may cause hyperuricaemia. The published prevalence of this abnormality is 13–42%, but controlled studies have shed some doubt on this metabolic association. Paget's disease and gout can clearly co-exist.

Radiological investigation

Plain radiographs either requested specifically to investigate the cause of bone pain, or serendipitously during other examinations, e.g. intravenous urogram, barium enema are important tools in the diagnosis of Paget's disease. The skeletal distribution of bone lesions varies between different

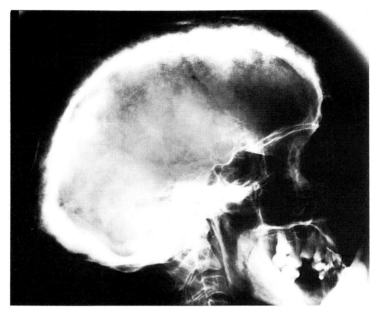

Fig. 4.7. Lateral radiograph of a Pagetic skull showing the frontal focal demineralisation of 'osteoporosis circumscripta'.

series but Table 4.3 indicates the approximate prevalence of bones
involved. Isotope bone scintigraphy (see below) is usually more sensitive
than plain radiography in defining Pagetic sites, and about 8% of lesions
will be missed by plain radiographic skeletal survey. In clinical practice, a
bone scintigram should be arranged soon after initial diagnosis of Paget's
disease to define affected bones and plain radiographs of these sites then
provide additional information. This protocol avoids the high radiation
exposure of the exhaustive skeletal survey.

Plain radiographs

Although the radiographic appearances of Paget's disease are very
distinctive, there is an 'infinite variety' of appearances. Some have claimed
that there is an ordered process of early osteolytic lesions followed by a
combined phase of osteolysis and sclerosis replaced, in turn, by a
dominantly sclerotic process. In practice mixed lesions are typical.

Marked osteolytic activity without an obviously adjacent sclerotic
response may be seen in the 'osteoporosis circumscripta of the skull (Fig.
4.7) or the V-shaped or flame-shaped advancing front in a long bone (Fig.

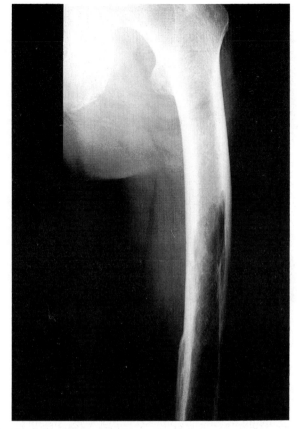

Fig. 4.8. Radiograph of the flame-shaped advancing front of Paget's disease in the femur. (By permission of Dr David Moore of Sheffield.)

4.8). More commonly radiographs demonstrate bony enlargement, cortical thickening, intracortical resorption, with a loss of cortico-medullary junction and accentuation of trabecular markings. Bowing deformities are common in long bones, and osteoarthritis is well defined by plain radiographs (Figs. 4.9 and 4.10). Hands are rarely affected (Fig. 4.11).

Isotope bone scintigraphy

Scintigraphy employing bone seeking isotopes such as ^{99}m Technetium-labelled polyphosphonates sensitively locate almost every Pagetic lesion, but there are exceptions. Occasional lesions proven by plain radiography fail to fix isotope suggesting the very rare occurrence of the 'burnt out' lesion and rarely, during aggressive advance of the resorption front,

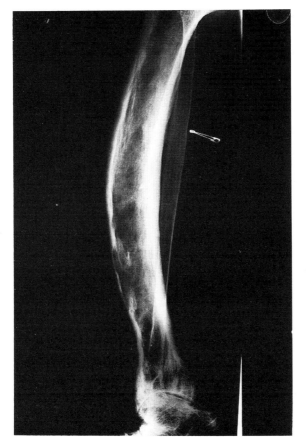

Fig. 4.9. Radiograph of a severely bowed tibia showing marked osteoarthritis of the ankle joint

scanning may underestimate disease activity. This implies that there is active osteoclastic resorption with a poor or absent osteoblastic response as bone scintigrams are revealing sites of new bone formation and not resorption. By the same mechanism, bone lesions in multiple myeloma are often missed by scintigraphy.

Typically, the bone scintigram in Paget's shows markedly increased uptake at affected sites and the pattern is only rarely confused with metastatic carcinoma, multiple fractures, osteomalacia or polyarthropathy, by the intensity of uptake (Fig. 4.12), and the distribution of lesions common in Paget's disease. A diagnostic problem sometimes occurs with a monostotic lesion, e.g. in the spine, and may need needle or open biopsy to prove the diagnosis. Bone scintigraphy is not very helpful in the

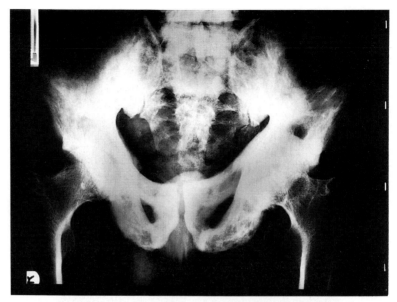

Fig. 4.10. Radiograph of the pelvis showing widespread Paget's disease and osteoarthritis of the left hip.

diagnosis of osteosarcoma in Paget's disease, although there may be decreased uptake at the malignant site.

There have been attempts to score the bone scintigram by quantitating uptake in affected areas and this correlates with biochemical indices of disease activity. Measurement of the whole body retention of isotope usually 24 hours after injection also gives a quantitative index of disease activity but is dependent on renal function. The reduction in whole body retention of isotope after treatment often seems unimpressive when compared with biochemical indices which is not easily understood.

Thermography

Increased bone and periosseous blood flow is demonstrated effectively in superficial bones and is reduced after effective treatment. Thermographic improvement and pain reduction seem to be linked.

Differential diagnosis of Paget's disease

The combination of physical signs including a warm deformed bone with characteristic radiographs and a raised serum alkaline phosphatase usually

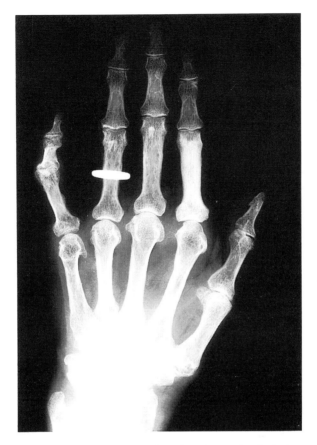

Fig. 4.11. Hand radiograph showing the sclerotic proximal phalanx of Paget's disease.

leaves no doubt about the diagnosis of Paget's disease, but it is worth considering.

1. Other causes of raised serum bone alkaline phosphatase (Table 4.5)
2. Other causes with a similar radiographic appearance (Table 4.6)

A detailed consideration of these diseases is outside the scope of this book, but it provides a fruitful area for discussion between clinician and radiologist and occasionally pathologist.

Treatment

Access to several safe and effective drugs for Paget's disease has led to earlier intervention with a wider range of indications for treatment than

Table. 4.5. *Causes of increased serum bone*
alkaline phosphatase

Paget's disease
Metastatic bone disease and bone tumours
Fractures   • trauma
                 • osteoporosis (transient)
Osteomalacia
Hyperparathyroidism with osteitis fibrosa cystica
Idiopathic hyperphosphatasia

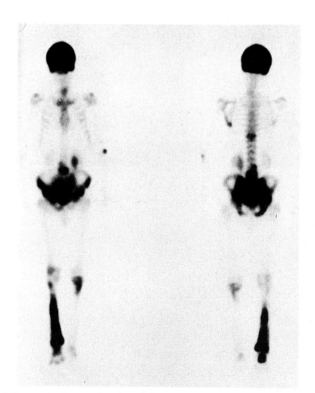

Fig. 4.12. A bone scintigram showing the typical appearance of widespread Paget's disease. (By permission of Oxford University Press: chapter by A.J. Crisp, *Oxford Textbook of Rheumatology.*)

Table. 4.6. *Differential diagnosis of Paget's disease – diseases with a similar radiological appearance*

Widespread osteosclerosis

Metastatic bone disease, especially prostate
Renal osteodystrophy
Myelosclerosis
Fluorosis
Hyperphosphatasia
Engelmann's disease (diaphyseal dysplasia)
Osteopetrosis
Fibrogenesis imperfecta
Pycnodystostosis
Polyostotic fibrous dysplasia

Focal osteosclerosis
Metastatic bone disease
Renal osteodystrophy
Haemangioma
Bone infarcts
Fibrous dysplasia
Chronic osteomyelitis
Lymphoma
Sternocostoclavicular hyperostosis
Melorheostosis
Osteopetrosis
Radiation osteitis

before (Table 4.7). Until recently some considered the sole indication for specific treatment was pain unresponsive to conventional analgesics, but the trend is now steadily towards early aggressive treatment with the intention of modifying the natural history of the disease and preventing complications of Paget's disease. It is argued that normalisation of serum alkaline phosphatase is now the goal of treatment as the duration of biochemical and clinical remission is related to the degree of biochemical improvement. There is strong histological evidence that effective disease control promotes more normal bone remodelling. However, it must be clearly stated that we lack firm evidence that intensive treatment affects long-term complications.

Pagetic and related osteoarthritic pain may be reduced by simple analgesics and non-steroidal anti-inflammatory drugs. Physical treatment with physiotherapy to improve muscle function and maintain mobility must be considered in all patients. Correcting inequalities in leg length with shoe raises can sometimes abolish knee or hip pain without recourse to

Table. 4.7. *Indications for treatment of Paget's disease*

Pain arising from a site of known Paget's disease
Early potentially deforming disease
Osteolytic lesions especially in weight-bearing bones
Skull involvement
Complications:

  Progressive neurological syndromes
  Fissure fractures (avoid etidronate)
  Immobilisation hypercalcaemia
  High output cardiac failure

Symptomatic or asymptomatic disease in patients under 55 years
Increase in serum alkaline phosphatase or urine hydroxyproline to twice
  maximum normal value

drugs. The rheumatologist is often the physician whose expertise in these physical and pharmacological areas is most appropriate.

Most patients with Paget's disease will at some stage require treatment with specific drugs, and their management is most appropriately planned by a specialist with an interest in musculo-skeletal medicine. The precise identity of that specialist will depend on local circumstances, but he is likely to be a rheumatologist, geriatrician or metabolic physician with a special interest in this field. The available drugs will first be discussed and then a practical management plan will be proposed.

The calcitonins

Calcitonin is a 32-amino acid polypeptide with a molecular weight of 3.5 kilodaltons. The endogenous hormone is produced by the parafollicular cells of the thyroid, and about 13 units are produced daily in man. Its major action is to reduce serum calcium and it remains uncertain whether endogenous calcitonin secretion is an important protector of the skeleton in situations when it is stressed, e.g. pregnancy and lactation, hyper-parathyroidism.

Several pharmacological preparations of calcitonin are available: salmon, porcine, eel and human. Salmon calcitonin (salcatonin) is the most widely used and is conventionally administered by the subcutaneous or intra-muscular route. Inhaled forms are very near to the market and work on oral preparations continues. There are differences in the potency of preparations: salmon and eel formulations are more potent in man than human or porcine hormone.

Calcitonin inhibits bone resorption (and turnover) by a direct action on the osteoclast which exhibits calcitonin receptors. It inhibits the activity and number of osteoclasts both in vitro and in vivo. Calcitonin was first used successfully in the treatment of Paget's disease in the 1960s. It has an early effect on bone resorption as reflected by reduced urine hydroxyproline excretion followed by a later fall in alkaline phosphatase by the usual coupling mechanisms of bone resorption and formation. Calcitonin can clearly halt the advance of the resorption front, increase bone mass by inhibition of bone remodelling and lead to replacement of woven bone by lamellar bone. It seems to have an early, rapid effect on bone blood flow and cardiac output within a few days of administration, and before any significant effect on bone turnover.

Dosage regimens of salcatonin vary from 100–200 units daily to 50 units three times weekly. Often treatment is started with 100 units daily subcutaneously following a 10 unit test dose (to detect the rare allergic response) for 1–3 months until a satisfactory therapeutic response has been achieved. This is followed by a maintenance regimen of 50–100 three times weekly. Patients are often taught to administer their own injections. Human and porcine calcitonins are less potent and far less widely used than salcatonin.

Serum alkaline phosphatase and urine hydroxyproline usually fall to 40–50% of pre-treatment value over 4–12 months, but frequently normalisation of alkaline phosphatase is not achieved and a 'plateau response' is noted. Sometimes, in spite of continuing treatment, there is the 'escape' of the increasing alkaline phosphatase level, and these phenomena have been explained on the basis of either upregulation of the calcitonin receptor (causing cellular 'resistance' to the effect of the hormone), or to the presence of circulating antibodies to calcitonin. Calcitonin resistance probably occurs in about 20% of patients.

Certainly if calcitonin is stopped, disease activity increases rapidly and there is still argument over the appropriate duration of treatment. Calcitonin is very safe and is still probably the treatment of first choice in the United States. Unpleasant, but not serious, side-effects are common: nausea, flushing, vomiting, diarrhoea, and pain at the site of injection. These are minimised by use of the subcutaneous route with injections given at bedtime.

Calcitonin administered by nasal spray is likely to become available in the United Kingdom during 1993. Doses of 400 units daily seem to be effective.

The bisphosphonates

This family of pyrophosphate analogues share a common P-C-P backbone, replacing the P-O-P of pyrophosphate. Side-chain variations confer

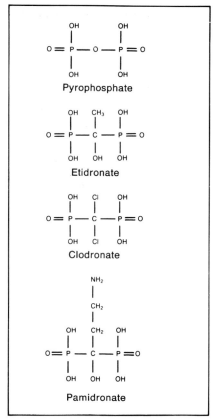

Fig. 4.13. The structures of pyrophosphate and of some bisphosphonates.

differing properties but they are all effective for Pagetic pain and disease activity (Fig. 4.13). The only example licensed for the treatment of Paget's disease in the United Kingdom is etidronate, but there is increasing experience with pamidronate and clodronate, which are at present licensed only for use in malignant hypercalcaemia. Further compounds undergoing evaluation include dimethylpamidronate, tiludronate and risedronate.

Bisphosphonates are poorly absorbed by mouth and are best taken on an empty stomach. They have a high affinity for bone. They are primary inhibitors of bone resorption and have an early suppressive effect on urine hydroxyproline excretion reflecting this. Formation falls later by the coupling process. There may be differences between the bisphosphonates in their precise mode of action on, e.g. osteoclast differentiation, rather than on the actively resorbing mature cell, but broadly these drugs are similar, varying in potency, gut absorption characteristics, and in their ability to inhibit bone mineralisation. Bisphosphonates trigger a mild secondary

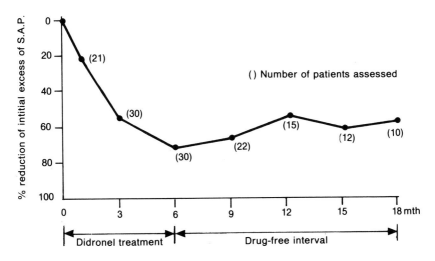

In a 51 patient study, Didronel was administered at
5mg/kg/day for 6 months

Fig. 4.14. The effect of oral etidronate (Didronel) on serum alkaline phosphatase
in Paget's disease. (By permission of Alexandre, C.M. *et al.*, 1983.)

hyperparathyroidism but this is unlikely to be of much practical clinical
significance.

Etidronate

Etidronate is given by mouth at a conventional dose of 5 mg/kg/day for 6
months, although a month's course of 20 mg/kg/day is probably as effective
without added toxicity (Fig. 4.14). The limiting factor with etidronate (in
contrast to later generation bisphosphonates) is the risk of demineralisation which can increase the risk of pathological fracture through Pagetic
long bones. If a dose of 5 mg/kg/day for 6 months, or 10 mg/kg/day for 3
months is used, the chances of developing a significant mineralisation
defect are minimal but this is almost universal if a dose as high as 20
mg/kg/day for 6 months is rashly employed.

   If the regimen of 20 mg/kg/day for 1 month is used, mineralisation is
rapidly impaired, but this is reversed when treatment is stopped. This will
achieve a satisfactory clinical response in most patients for about a year or
more, when the course may be repeated as judged by a return of symptoms
and a climbing alkaline phosphatase. This represents a marked advantage
over calcitonin when relapse is rapid after treatment ceases.

   With the exception of the mineralisation defect which occurs if too high a dose is employed for too long, etidronate is very safe. Mild gastrointestinal symptoms, such as diarrhoea, and transient increase in bone pain can occur, but are rarely severe enough to discontinue treatment. Etidronate is probably wisely avoided in patients with extensive osteolytic lesions of long bones and with fissure fractures although this may be an over-cautious view.

Pamidronate

Pamidronate is up to 20 times more potent than etidronate. It is highly effective in both oral and intravenous forms and treatment failure, as judged by changes in bone pain and alkaline phosphatase, is rare if appropriate doses are employed. In the United Kingdom, pamidronate is only available in the intravenous formulation and, it should be emphasised, is only licensed for use in malignant hypercalcaemia.

There is, however, a considerable experience of its use in Paget's disease and it has become an important treatment in centres with a special interest in the disease. There remains no consensus on the optimal dose regimen which varies from 500 mg orally daily to intravenous regimens of 15 mg daily for 5 days to 30 mg weekly for 12 weeks. The most promising development has been the use of single intravenous infusions of higher doses such as 60–105 mg which have been shown to achieve an excellent clinical and biochemical remission for up to 2 years with equally successful retreatments after that (Fig. 4.15).

Gastrointestinal side-effects suggest that pamidronate may not be widely used in the future by the oral route. Transient fever and clinically insignificant leucopenia are common side-effects with no known long-term sequelae so far noted. Fever does not return after retreatment. A transient increase in hydroxyproline excretion may occur paradoxically after pamidronate, perhaps stimulated by interleukins 1 and 6 release which are known to stimulate bone resorption. The bone demineralisation defect caused by etidronate has not been reported with pamidronate.

Clodronate

Experience with clodronate has been comparable with that of pamidronate. In the United Kingdom, this is available in oral and intravenous forms which are licensed for use only in malignant hypercalcaemia. Clodronate 1600 mg daily for one month by mouth or 300 mg intravenously daily for 5 days seem to achieve equivalent results with a prolonged clinical and biochemical improvement without a secondary mineralisation defect. The acceptance of clodronate has been slowed by the report of three cases of

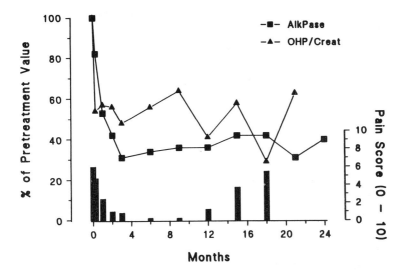

Fig. 4.15. The effect of pamidronate 105 mg intravenously on biochemical indices and pain in seven patients with Paget's disease. Note the rapid initial fall in urine hydroxyproline/creatinine ratio (OHP/creat) and the slightly delayed fall in serum alkaline phosphatase. Pain is typically well controlled for at least a year with gradual relapse in the second year. It is recommended that single infusion treatment should usually be restricted to 60 mg doses.

leukaemia in patients who had received this drug, but it is now widely accepted that this association was coincidental.

Mithramycin (plicamycin)

This is a cytotoxic antibiotic which inhibits RNA synthesis. It has been used in Paget's disease with intravenous doses of 10–25 µg/kg/day for 7–10 days with great effect. Remissions are typically short but occasionally are prolonged. Its use is limited by hepatic, renal and bone marrow toxicity, and can now only rarely be justified with the advent of newer bisphosphonates. It may still be useful for selected patients with severe disease, and for those requiring a rapid response as in progressive paraplegia.

The practical management of the patient with Paget's disease

Most patients prefer to accept specific treatment for their disease rather than just analgesics, although these can be useful especially while awaiting the effect of bisphosphonates or calcitonin. Review by a physiotherapist will often give some practical tips, such as the use of a heel raise, as well as improve the patient's morale by teaching a programme of self-help exercises.

Oral etidronate is likely to be the drug of first choice, employing a course of either 10 mg/kg/day for 3 months, or 20 mg/kg/day for 1 month. This is likely to be effective treatment in 70–80% of patients and the intention should be to reduce alkaline phosphatase to or near to the normal range.

It is wise to allow a generous treatment-free interval between courses to allow healing of any possible mineralisation defect. If the clinical response is unsatisfactory, then it is worth considering a course of salcatonin 100 units daily for 2–3 months following a 10 unit test dose, with a maintenance dose of 50 units 3 times weekly for a further 3–6 months, depending on response. If the salcatonin course achieves a satisfactory remission, then it is worth trying to maintain this with further oral courses of etidronate judged by a combination of symptoms and sequential alkaline phosphatase measurements.

If the patient has not responded effectively to this treatment approach with satisfactory control of pain and a normal or near-normal alkaline phosphatase, then referral to a centre with a special interest in Paget's disease is recommended for consideration of unlicensed treatment with pamidronate, clodronate or, rarely, with mithramycin.

There is still no consensus as to whether patients requiring total joint replacements or other orthopaedic surgery for the ravages of the combination of Paget's disease and osteoarthritis should receive specific medical treatment before surgery. There is a little evidence that effective treatment reduces bone blood flow, improves the quality of bone in which the prosthesis will be sited, and facilitates adhesion of cement to bone. Certainly, orthopaedic surgeons should not be deterred from replacement arthroplasty by the presence of Paget's disease as the risks of prosthetic loosening are only slightly increased. It would seem logical to time surgery to coincide with a phase of clinical and biochemical remission induced by medical treatment.

Further reading

Alexandre, C.M. *et al.* (1983). *Clinical Orthopaedics and Related Research*, **174**, 193–200.

Kanis, J.A. (1991). *Pathophysiology and Treatment of Paget's Disease of Bone*. Martin Dunitz, pp. 1–298.

5

The hypercalcaemic patient

Hypercalcaemia is common in both the general population and especially in hospital populations. During a 6-month period in Birmingham, all patients presenting with hypercalcaemia were studied. It was estimated that there are 270 new cases of primary hyperparathyroidism (the commonest cause of hypercalcaemia) and 150 new cases of malignant hypercalcaemia per million population every year. Similar incidence figures were obtained in the United States in epidemiological studies in Olmsted County, Minnesota. A wide range of diseases can cause hypercalcaemia (Table 5.1) but in clinical practice about 90% of cases are caused by primary hyperparathyroidism (54%) or malignancy (35%).

The clinical features of hypercalcaemia

The spectrum of symptoms and signs which can be caused by hypercalcaemia is vast (Table 5.2). Patients with mild disease are often asymptomatic, or suffer symptoms so mild that they are only recognised in retrospect after the correction of hypercalcaemia. A rapid increase in serum calcium and very high values are most likely to induce marked symptoms.

Neuropsychiatric features

Close relatives and friends may notice behavioural changes in patients with hypercalcaemia and the common clinical symptoms often offered to doctors of undue 'tiredness,' 'exhaustion' and 'lack of energy' demand a calcium estimation. Milder symptoms of headache and sleep disturbance may be followed by confusion as calcium concentrations increase and, if untreated, patients may deteriorate with progressive change in levels of consciousness. Sometimes, more bizarre psychiatric states can occur with

Table. 5.1. *The causes of hypercalcaemia*

Common	
Primary hyperparathyroidism	
Malignant disease	• humoral hypercalcaemia of malignancy
	• metastatic bone disease
	• multiple myeloma
Less common	
1. Other endocrine	• hyperthyroidism
	• Addison's disease
2. Iatrogenic or self-induced	• thiazide diuretics
	• vitamin D toxicity
	• vitamin A toxicity
	• excessive thyroxine replacement therapy
	• milk–alkali syndrome
3. Renal	• chronic renal failure
	• diuretic phase of acute renal failure
4. Other	• sarcoidosis and other granulomatous diseases
	• Paget's disease (rarely) especially if immobilised
	• immobilisation *per se* (especially younger patients)
	• familial hypocalciuric hypercalcaemia (FHH)

delusion or hallucination and physicians in neurological and psychiatric practice should have a low threshold for a serum calcium request.

Gastrointestinal features

Constipation, anorexia and vomiting are very frequent symptoms. The relationship with peptic ulceration remains controversial. Increased gastric acid and pepsin secretion has been demonstrated. Atropine can block calcium-stimulated gastric acid release suggesting a cholinergic nerve mechanism.

Acute pancreatitis is a rare, though well-documented, complication of hypercalcaemia especially with primary hyperparathyroidism. The mechanism is unknown.

Renal features

Hypercalcaemia reduces the ability of the kidney to concentrate urine causing polyuria, polydipsia and nocturia. It may inhibit the action of anti-diuretic hormone. Patients with primary hyperparathyroidism have a

Table. 5.2. *Clinical features of hypercalcaemia*

Neuropsychiatric	• lethargy
	• headache
	• confusion and disorientation
	• sleep disturbance
	• depression and irritability
	• altered level of consciousness • drowsiness
	                                          • stupor
	                                          • coma

Gastrointestinal	• anorexia • nausea and vomiting • constipation • acute pancreatitis • ? peptic ulceration
Renal	• polyuria • polydipsia • nocturia • hypercalciuria • nephrocalcinosis • reduced glomerular filtration rate
Cardiological	• arrhythmias • ? hypertension
Musculoskeletal	• arthralgia and arthritis • myalgia • hypotonia and muscle weakness • osteitis fibrosa cystica (primary hyperparathyroidism only)
Ophthalmic	• corneal calcification
Skin	• pruritus and skin necrosis

mild hyperchloraemic acidosis in contrast to the hypochloraemic alkalosis which occurs typically with other causes of hypercalcaemia. Hypercalcaemia may impair glomerular function, and also tubular function, most commonly in myeloma. Patients presenting with renal stones should always be investigated for hypercalciuria and hypercalcaemia.

Cardiological features

There is some evidence that hypercalcaemia causes hypertension by a vasoconstrictive effect on smooth muscle. Calcium infusions can elevate blood pressure which returns to normal after the infusion. EDTA, which reduces serum calcium, can decrease blood pressure.

Hypercalcaemia stimulates myocardial contractility and conduction.

The ECG may demonstrate shortening of the QT interval and widening of the T-wave. Severe hypercalcaemia can kill the patient by ventricular fibrillation or asystole. It should also be noted that calcium and digoxin have a synergistic effect and that digoxin should only be used with great caution in the presence of hypercalcaemia.

Musculoskeletal features

Non-specific aches and pains are common and a true inflammatory symmetrical polyarthritis has been recorded rarely with primary hyperparathyroidism. There is no association between rheumatoid arthritis and hyperparathyroidism but, when these two common conditions coexist, hypercalcaemia seems to exacerbate the arthritis. Following parathyroidectomy, the arthritis can remit.

The investigation of hypercalcaemia

A detailed history from the patient may identify the underlying cause of hypercalcaemia without recourse to further investigations beyond the serum calcium concentration. A background of a known relevant disease, the discovery of excessive self-medication with vitamin supplements or of thiazide medication will clearly determine that patient's management. More often the range of symptoms described and elicited will suggest that a serum calcium estimation would be well justified. Physical examination may add little to the clinical picture already painted by the history but some clues may be sought. The hypercalcaemic patient may be rather irritable and dislike the physical inconvenience of the examination. Perhaps only corneal calcification at the corneal–scleral junction often most marked at 3 and 9 o'clock is a specific physical sign of hypercalcaemia. It usually indicates chronic hypercalcaemia and therefore primary hyperparathyroidism.

If a history and examination have failed to determine the most likely cause of the hypercalcaemia, an appropriate protocol for investigation might include:

Blood   Full blood count
            Erythrocyte sedimentation rate (ESR)
            Urea and electrolytes
            Liver function tests
            Serum calcium, phosphate, alkaline phosphatase
            TSH, thyroxine
            Protein immunoelectrophoresis
            Serum intact parathyroid hormone (PTH)

Urine   24-hour urine collection for   • calcium
                                           • phosphate
                                           • creatinine clearance
          Early morning urine for Bence–Jones protein
Imaging   Chest radiograph
          Isotope bone scan
          Other imaging tests indicated by the patient's symptoms and signs

If the patient's condition is stable and satisfactory there is no indication to admit the patient to hospital. All of these tests can be performed in the outpatient clinic.

Serum calcium

Most laboratories provide a measurement of total serum calcium which comprises the free, active or 'ionised' calcium (about 47%) and the bound, inactive calcium. A total calcium measurement may not accurately reflect ionised calcium status. Inactive calcium is bound mainly to albumin. In the presence of low albumin values with liver disease, poor nutrition or other chronic diseases, the total serum calcium is therefore also low. Some calcium is also bound to globulins and, in hyperglobulinaemic states such as myeloma, the total serum calcium may be misleadingly raised. Alkalosis and acidosis reduce or increase the ionised calcium owing to changes in protein binding. Traditionally and with justification the total serum calcium concentration is 'corrected' for albumin concentration, the main serum factor influencing its measurement. One favoured correction is to add or subtract 0.02 mmol/l for every 1 g/l albumin below or above an albumin concentration of 40 g/l. For example, a total serum calcium of 2.64 mmol/l in the presence of albumin concentration of 38 g/l may be corrected to 2.68 mmol/l.

The absolute value of serum calcium does not aid in finding the underlying cause of hypercalcaemia. Most patients, irrespective of the cause, present with a serum calcium of less than 3.5 mmol/l. Both primary hyperparathyroidism and malignancy can cause high values more than 4.0 mmol/l.

Serum ionised calcium can be measured by an ion-selective electrode and is useful in cases of borderline total hypercalcaemia. Its measurement does not aid in differential diagnosis.

Serum phosphorus

This can vary considerably with diet, falling after a carbohydrate meal, and with age with higher values in childhood. Patients with primary hyperparathyroidism usually have decreased serum phosphate as PTH reduces renal tubular phosphate reabsorption. A similar change may occur in malignant hypercalcaemia and so it is unhelpful as a distinguishing test. Diseases causing increased gastrointestinal calcium absorption, e.g. sarcoidosis and vitamin D toxicity, also tend to increase serum phosphate. The formal measurement of tubular maximal reabsorption of phosphate related to glomerular filtration rate (TMP/GFR) is of little value.

Serum chloride and bicarbonate

Many laboratories no longer offer serum chloride measurements routinely but patients with primary hyperparathyroidism usually have a serum chloride of more than 103 mmol/l (metabolic acidosis) and patients with hypercalcaemia of malignancy usually have a value less than 100 mmol/l.

Serum alkaline phosphatase

This osteoblast-derived enzyme is often increased in patients with more than mild hyperparathyroidism and in patients with most forms of malignant hypercalcaemia. Patients with myeloma and some lymphomas with bone involvement often have a normal serum alkaline phosphatase because of a poor or absent bone formation response to malignant bone loss.

Serum immunoreactive PTH

PTH radioimmunoassays remain imperfect tools, but have become more reliable recently. There is often a dissociation between the immunoreactivity in assays of PTH fragments and their biological action. Recent assays utilising antibodies directed at two different sites on the PTH molecule, both the N-terminal and C-terminal ends ('intact PTH assays') are a major advance and more reliably distinguish between primary hyperparathyroidism and hypercalcaemia of malignancy (caused by PTH related protein-PTHrP, see later).

In spite of technical improvements in PTH assays primary hyperparathyroidism is not necessarily excluded by a value in the mid or upper range of normal when interpreted alongside significant hypercalcaemia. Clinical judgement based on clinical and laboratory evidence is still important.

Vitamin D metabolites

Serum 25-hydroxyvitamin D is widely measured and reflects vitamin D intake. It will prove a suspected diagnosis of vitamin D toxicity.

Serum 1,25-dihydroxyvitamin D measurement is less widely available but may be increased in primary hyperparathyroidism as its synthesis is stimulated by PTH. This vitamin D metabolite can also be synthesised in extra-renal sites in sarcoidosis and other granulomatous diseases. Rarely, it is increased in patients with hypercalcaemia caused by T and B cell lymphomas and Hodgkin's disease.

Urine studies

Urine calcium excretion is normal or increased in virtually all patients with hypercalcaemia and does not help to discriminate between alternative diagnoses. Hypercalciuria will predispose to renal stone formation and nephrocalcinosis. Urine calcium measurements are of most critical use in the diagnosis of familial hypocalciuric hypercalcaemia when calcium excretion is reduced. It is worth considering in patients with apparent primary hyperparathyroidism who are young and often asymptomatic. It is an autosomal dominant disorder.

Measurements of urine phosphate and creatinine on the same 24-hour specimen will help to assess the completeness of the collection and also glomerular function. Urine cyclic AMP measurements once fashionable for diagnosing primary hyperparathyroidism are poor discriminants and are now only rarely made. A concentrated morning urine specimen for Bence-Jones protein will with serum protein immunoelectrophoresis aid the diagnosis of myeloma.

Imaging studies

A chest radiograph will demonstrate relevant malignant disease and sarcoidosis, and is always worthwhile. A small number of patients with primary hyperparathyroidism, now that the diagnosis is made at an earlier stage, will have the typical radiological changes of osteitis fibrosa cystica (Fig. 5.1 and 5.2) [see later]. A limited skeletal survey may suggest the diagnosis of myeloma.

An isotope bone scan is often very helpful. It should demonstrate metastatic bone disease but may overlook myelomatous bone involvement because of the poor or absent osteoblastic response, on which bone

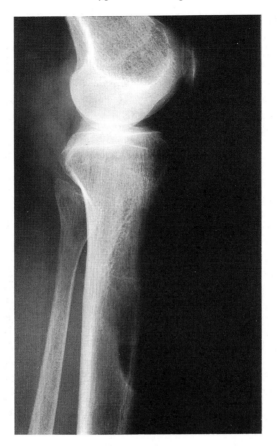

Fig. 5.1. A lateral view of the knee in severe primary hyperparathyroidism showing the extensive erosion of bone in the proximal tibia and replacement by fibrous tissue [the 'brown tumour'] of osteitis fibrosa cystica. (By courtesy of Dr David Moore of Sheffield.)

scintigraphy relies. A bone scan may reveal areas which should be investigated further with plain radiographs or computerised tomography.

The corticosteroid suppression test

This test was developed by Charles Dent of University College Hospital, London, before the arrival of reliable PTH immunoassays and it is still occasionally useful in the discrimination between primary hyper-parathyroidism and other causes of hypercalcaemia. Prednisolone 10 mg every 8 hours, or hydrocortisone 40 mg every 8 hours by mouth for 10 days

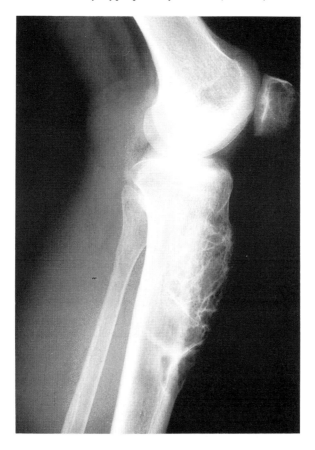

Fig. 5.2. A lateral view of the same knee as in Fig. 5.1 showing the partial healing of the 'brown tumour' after parathyroidectomy. (By courtesy of Dr David Moore of Sheffield.)

fails to suppress hypercalcaemia in primary hyperparathyroidism but is successful in almost all other patients. Occasionally, the hypercalcaemia of malignancy is not suppressed.

Primary hyperparathyroidism (PHPT)

PHPT is caused by excess and inappropriate PTH production by one or more of the parathyroid glands in the neck. The first clinical description of the disease was by Mandl in 1926. He described a 39 year-old Viennese bus conductor with deformities of the pelvis, femur, and knee with marked bone softening. Mandl initially interpreted this as parathyroid gland

Table. 5.3. *Multiple endocrine neoplasia [MEN]*

Type I	Primary hyperparathyroidism
	Pituitary adenoma • acromegaly
	• prolactinoma
	Pancreatic adenoma
Type II	Primary hyperparathyroidism
	Phaeochromocytoma
	Medullary carcinoma of the thyroid
	Mucosal neuroma (occasionally)

deficiency but later removed either a parathyroid adenoma or a hyperplastic gland with dramatic clinical improvement. The disease, considered to be a rare, esoteric metabolic phenomenon was popularised by Fuller Albright, a physician at Massachusetts General Hospital, Boston, who collected large numbers of these patients with 'bones, stones and abdominal groans.' We now know that PHPT is a common disease with about 270 new cases a year per million of population, and a prevalance of about 0.1%.

Pathology

PHPT may be caused by:

(a) a solitary parathyroid gland adenoma (85%)
(b) hyperplasia of all four glands (almost 15%)
(c) carcinoma of a parathyroid gland (very rare)

Most adenomas are composed of the chief cells and sometimes of cells 'transitional' between chief and oxyphil cells. A normal gland weighs 25–50 mg and adenomas can weigh up to 20 g. The inferior glands are most often involved but in about 5–10% of cases the gland is sited abnormally in the thymus, thyroid, mediastinum, pericardium, or retro-oesophageal space. Chief cell hyperplasia of all four glands is much less common. The clinical presentation is identical. Carcinoma of the parathyroid gland is very rare. Less than 200 cases have been reported. Hypercalcaemia is usually more severe. Local invasion and recurrence of the malignant tumour is more common than metastasis.

PHPT may occur in association with multiple endocrine neoplasia (MEN) Types I and II (Table 5.3).

Aetiology

Single parathyroid gland adenomas are likely to be a monoclonal disorder arising from an abnormality in a single cell. Hyperplasia is likely to be the

Table. 5.4. *Skeletal involvement in
primary hyperparathyroidism*

Osteoporosis
Sub-periosteal resorption
Osteosclerosis
Loss of lamina dura
Cystic lesions   • 'brown tumours'
• true bone cysts

result of less defined stimuli perhaps related to fibroblast growth factors (FGF) released in response to chronic hypocalcaemia. Previous neck irradiation has been implicated in the aetiology. Common to all forms is the inappropriate release of PTH which is no longer controlled by serum calcium concentration.

Clinical features

The clinical features of hypercalcaemia have already been described at the start of this Chapter and they are typical of PHPT. Earlier studies emphasised the involvement of bone and the high frequency of renal stones. In one large British series in 1974, 47% of the patients presented with renal stones and nephrocalcinosis and 13% with bone involvement. In contrast in another British study a decade later, 51% of patients with PHPT were asymptomatic or discovered accidentally. Only 6% had renal involvement. Clearly local referral patterns will determine the nature of the affected population.

Some specific features of PHPT deserve further attention.

Skeletal features (Table 5.4)

Although skeletal involvement is now relatively rare in PHPT owing to earlier diagnosis and treatment, osteitis fibrosa cystica is pathognonomic of PHPT (Figs. 5.1 and 5.2). Generalised bone loss caused by the effect of elevated PTH on the skeleton and now more easily demonstrated by bone densitometry is now probably more common. Thus patients now present with vertebral crush fractures rather than long bone deformity. Histologically, as the name implies, osteitis fibrosa cystica is characterised by increased osteoclastic bone resorption, increased osteoblastic new bone formation and by sometimes striking peritrabecular marrow fibrosis.

Skeletal radiographs are probably normal in more than 80% of cases of

PHPT. In a minority, therefore, osteopenia, subperiosteal resorption of bone (radiological hallmark of osteitis fibrosa cystica), osteosclerosis, loss of the lamina dura of the teeth and cystic lesions may be identified. Subperiosteal bone resorption is most easily identified in the phalanges, acromioclavicular joint, symphysis pubis and sacroiliac joints. The radial aspect of the middle phalanges and the tufts of the terminal phalanges are classically involved. A mottled skull appearance and tapering of the distal third of the clavicles are also characteristic. Osteosclerosis may occur in 5–20% of patients with secondary hyperparathyroidism secondary to chronic renal failure and is very rare in PHPT. The paradoxical anabolic effect of PTH on the skeleton, exploited in experimental treatments for osteoporosis, is probably responsible. The 'brown tumours' of PHPT are cellular and represent osteoclastomas. They resolve after parathyroid surgery unlike the bone cysts which can also occur.

Neuromuscular features

A specific atrophy of the Type II muscle fibres of neuropathic origin has been described in PHPT. Clinically it is characterised by weakness and easy fatiguability, proximal muscle wasting and normal serum muscle enzyme concentrations. Mild versions of this syndrome may be common.

Articular features

The most frequently seen articular complication of PHPT is pyrophosphate arthropathy (Fig. 5.3). Up to 18% of patients with PHPT may be affected by this disorder. It is characterised by calcification of articular cartilage (chondrocalcinosis) and by the clinical syndrome of pseudogout in which patients suffer recurrent attacks of inflammatory monoarthritis or polyarthritis. Parathyroidectomy may precipitate acute attacks which can continue to occur long after surgery and the achievement of normocalcaemia. Joint fluid aspirated from the inflamed joint may reveal the positively birefringent crystals of calcium pyrophosphate. Hyperuricaemia and its clinical consequence, acute gout, also occurs in PHPT owing to the reduced renal clearance of urate.

Subchondral fractures caused by bone softening leading to a secondary synovitis and calcific periarthritis have also been described. Spontaneous quadriceps muscle–tendon junction avulsions are also said to occur.

Pregnancy and childhood

Severe neonatal hypocalcaemia can occur with the prolonged suppression of PTH secretion which occurs as a consequence of maternal hypercalcaemia. Pregnant women with severe hypercalcaemia should therefore

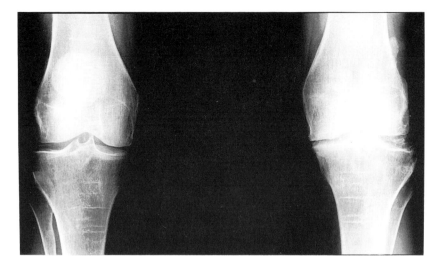

Fig. 5.3. AP radiographs of knees from a patient with primary hyper-parathyroidism. Note the calcifications of the articular cartilage and menisci (chondrocalcinosis).

probably undergo parathyroidectomy before delivery. PHPT is rare in childhood. It is always important to exclude familial hypocalciuric hypercalcaemia.

'Parathyroid crisis'

Rarely patients (usually elderly) with PHPT may present with fever, dehydration, altered level of consciousness and a marked increase in serum calcium to high levels (more than 4.5 mmol/l). Untreated it can be fatal. It is worth considering in all patients presenting in a 'shock-like' state.

Multiple endocrine neoplasia (MEN)

MEN Type I (Table 5.3) may account for up to 10% of patients with PHPT and is always worth considering. MEN Type II is less common and usually comes to light after the diagnosis of medullary carcinoma of the thyroid as most patients are normocalcaemic.

The treatment of primary hyperparathyroidism

Probably more than half the patients in whom a diagnosis of PHPT is made are asymptomatic and the first decision is whether any treatment is

Table. 5.5. *Indications for parathyroidectomy in primary hyperparathyroidism*

1.	Symptoms or signs caused by hypercalcaemia or primary hyperparathyroidism
2.	Patients who are inaccessible to long-term follow-up
3.	Corrected serum calcium more than 2.9 mmol/l
4.	Parathyroid carcinoma

necessary. Many of these patients will remain asymptomatic for many years. It is not difficult to elicit a history of mild symptoms in many patients, for example, constipation, tiredness and headache but it is not always apparent that these can be linked to PHPT. A large prospective study from the Mayo Clinic of 134 patients suggested that over half of these asymptomatic patients remained asymptomatic over 5 years.

In Table 5.5 one set of criteria for surgical parathyroidectomy is listed. The availability of a specialist neck surgeon well experienced in parathyroid surgery, many would consider, is an equally important criterion.

Management of the asymptomatic patient

These patients deserve a full assessment for evidence of subclinical disease including careful investigation of renal function and bone involvement. A baseline measurement of bone density may also be useful so that the rate of future bone loss can be calculated. Patients with PHPT may not necessarily continue to lose bone but evidence of accelerated loss would probably require surgical intervention. Outpatient review every 6 months is appropriate to detect evidence of renal deterioration or other clinical involvement. Annual measurements of bone density are desirable.

Medical treatment

Long-term medical treatment for PHPT is not very satisfactory. Oral phosphate in doses up to 2 g/day and only in patients with low normal serum concentrations of phosphate can help to control mild hypercalcaemia. Phosphate, however, often causes diarrhoea.

Later generation bisphosphonates, e.g. pamidronate and clodronate, have been used successfully and are of great use in patients with hypercalcaemia caused by parathyroid carcinoma. Oestrogen therapy also seems to be effective without influencing PTH concentration in post-menopausal women.

Treatment of 'parathyroid crisis' with severe hypercalcaemia is with rehydration, subcutaneous salcatonin and probably with intravenous pamidronate or clodronate in addition (for specific details of management, see also 'Emergency treatment for malignant hypercalcaemia' p. 139). Corticosteroids are usually ineffective in the presence of hyper-parathyroidism.

Surgical treatment

Surgery is the definitive treatment for PHPT. The indications for surgery are listed in Table 5.5. A procedure to localise the parathyroid adenoma is usually not indicated at the first neck exploration. Hyperplasia (in 15% of cases) should be suspected in those patients with a family history of MEN. In 5–10% of cases the adenoma may be in an ectopic site. Surgery requires a surgeon particularly experienced in parathyroid disease and a pathologist who will examine frozen sections removed at surgery. It is easy to confuse parathyroid tissue with fat or lymph nodes and all four glands should be identified. A single adenoma should be excised. If parathyroid hyperplasia of all four glands is found, then 3½ glands should be excised. If an adenoma is not found, the surgeon examines the retro-oesophageal and retro-pharyngeal spaces and tissue around the thymus.

If pathological parathyroid tissue cannot be identified at surgery, localisation procedures are usually undertaken with ultrasound, computed tomography, thallium or MIBI scintigraphy. Selective venous sampling, and then submitting the samples to PTH assay, is now only very rarely required.

The most common post-operative complication is hypocalcaemia and this usually occurs in patients with bone disease (the 'hungry bone syndrome'). It may be profound and need high doses of vitamin D to maintain normocalcaemia. Hypocalcaemia may continue as a result of inadequate functional parathyroid tissue remaining after surgery. It is most likely in patients with hyperplasia who have undergone removal of 3½ glands. These patients need lifelong treatment with oral calcium and vitamin D, but this decision should not be made until 6 months after surgery as gland recovery can occur up to this stage. The doses are judged by frequent monitoring of serum calcium.

Table. 5.6. *Malignancies associated
with hypercalaemia (%)*

Lung	35
Breast	25
Haematological (myeloma, lymphoma)	14
Head and neck	6
Renal	3
Prostate	3
Unknown primary	7
Others	8

Table. 5.7. *Malignancies frequently
associated with humoral
hypercalcaemia of malignancy (HHM)*

Squamous carcinoma of the lung, head and neck
Carcinoma of the kidney
Carcinoma of the ovary
Carcinoma of the pancreas

Malignant hypercalcaemia

Malignancy is the cause of about 35% of cases with hypercalcaemia and the types of disease are listed in Table 5.6. Malignant causes of hypercalcaemia are likely to be over-represented in a hospital population as the patients tend to be more ill than patients with PHPT. Some common carcinomas such as gynaecological tumours and colon only very rarely cause hypercalcaemia but some rare malignancies commonly cause it, cholangio carcinoma and VIPomas of the pancreas. There are three broad categories of malignant hypercalcaemia:
1. Humoral hypercalcaemia of malignancy [HHM]
2. Osteolytic metastases
3. Haematological malignancy, myeloma most commonly

Each category will be considered in turn.

Humoral hypercalcaemia of malignancy [HHM]

This occurs in patients with solid tumours most commonly carcinoma of the bronchus in whom circulating humoral factors cause hypercalcaemia (Table 5.7). They may, or may not, have focal bone metastases.

Pathophysiology

There is strong evidence of increased osteoclastic bone resorption, increased renal tubular calcium reabsorption and reduced absorption of calcium from the gut. Other features include normal or decreased plasma immunoreactive PTH, reduced or low normal 1,25 dihydroxyvitamin D concentrations and mild hypochloraemic metabolic alkalosis.

Many of these features suggested that PTH or a PTH-like substance was playing a major role in pathogenesis but increased concentrations of PTH by radioimmunoassay could not be consistently demonstrated. The terms 'pseudohyperparathyroidism' or 'ectopic PTH' syndrome were coined but really concealed ignorance. Eventually the cause of these hypercalcaemic syndromes was found to be 'PTH-related protein' (PTHrP). It has considerable amino acid sequence homology with authentic PTH-8 of the first 13 amino acids are identical in the portion which binds to the PTH receptor.

However, PTHrP is probably not the final complete answer in HHM. It is likely that its actions on larger organs are modified by other cytokines such as interleukin-1 (IL-1), transforming growth factor-alpha (TGFα) and tumour necrosis factors (TNF). These are all known to have potent effects on bone in vitro and act synergistically with PTH.

In addition to a direct effect on bone, the factors mediating HHM also promote hypercalcaemia both by reducing glomerular filtration and by increasing renal tubular reabsorption of calcium.

Diagnosis of HHM

Usually evidence of the underlying malignancy is clear. Uncommonly a patient with hypercalcaemia may have an occult malignancy. More commonly a patient with a malignancy may develop hypercalcaemia. PHPT may co-exist with malignancy and evidence for this may be obtained by the findings of:

- increased serum PTH
- hyperchloraemic acidosis
- renal phosphate wasting

In future it is hoped that access to reliable assays for PTHrP, TGF, IL-1 and TNF will make the diagnosis of HHM easier.

Management of HHM

Complete removal of the underlying tumour is the ideal. More commonly this is not possible and treatment is based on:

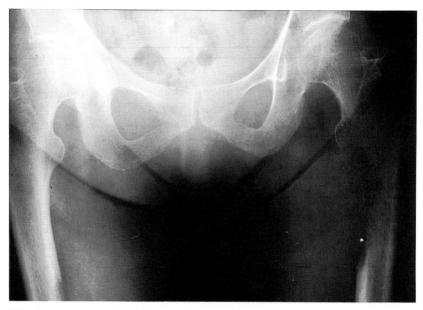

Fig. 5.4. Radiograph of femora in a patient with metastatic carcinoma of bronchus. Note the areas of bone resorption in both femora. (By courtesy of Dr David Moore of Sheffield.)

(a) rehydration and drugs which increase renal calcium excretion such as loop diuretics.

(b) drugs which inhibit bone resorption such as mithramycin (plicamycin), bisphosphonates, calcitonin and glucocorticoids.
(see later)

Osteolytic metastases and hypercalcaemia

Many tumours metastasise to bone, notoriously, breast, bronchus, prostate, kidney and thyroid, but breast cancer accounts for 25% of all cases of malignant hypercalcaemia (Fig. 5.4). The most common sites of bone metastases are, in decreasing order, the thoraco-columbar spine, pelvis, lower limbs, upper limbs and skull. The majority of bone metastases from breast cancer are osteolytic but about one-fifth are osteosclerotic as classically observed in prostate cancer. The appearance of hypercalcaemia in a patient with metastatic bone disease is usually a near terminal event. It is possible that humoral factors resorbing bone are also playing a part but this section is devoted to the process of direct resorption of bone by tumour itself. About 10–30% of patients with breast cancer develop hypercalcaemia usually at a late stage. About 90% of patients dying with breast cancer have bone metastases but metastases do not, of course, inevitably cause hypercalcaemia. The mean survival after diagnosis of hypercalcaemia in these patients is 3 months. Hypercalcaemia and bone lesions are more common in oestrogen-receptor positive tumours.

The mechanism of bone destruction in breast cancer is complex. Hypercalcaemia is mainly secondary to bone resorption but there is also a contribution from increased renal tubular reabsorption of calcium. There is still debate whether bone is directly resorbed by tumour cells or indirectly resorbed by production of local osteoclast activating factors stimulated by tumour or other cells. A full discussion of these issues is inappropriate here but the evidence has been well reviewed by Mundy (1990).

Hypercalcaemia associated with haematological malignancies

Myeloma is by far the most common haematological malignancy to cause hypercalcaemia and 20–40% of patients with myeloma develop hypercalcaemia at some stage in their disease.

Pathophysiology

Hypercalcaemia in myeloma is caused by a combination of increased bone resorption and irreversibly reduced glomerular filtration, which causes reduced renal calcium excretion. The bone lesions of myeloma which are almost universal in late disease have several distinct patterns:

(a) discrete osteolytic lesions by deposits of myeloma cells in the skeleton;
(b) diffuse osteopenia when myeloma cells are spread diffusely throughout the skeleton;
(c) discrete osteolytic lesions caused by plasmacytomas.

The underlying mechanism of bone loss is the stimulation of osteoclastic bone resorption by close proximity to myeloma cells and the inhibition of the osteoblastic attempts to reform bone in response to resorption. The failure of the isotope bone scan to demonstrate lesions and the classically normal alkaline phosphatase (in spite of a considerable increase in bone turnover) supports this concept of osteoblast inhibition. There are exceptions, e.g. after fracture, when an osteoblast response may be mounted.

Osteoclast activating factor or factors were described with activity distinct from other known bone resorbing hormones or mediators (PTH, prostaglandins, vitamin D metabolites). Likely candidates are interleukin-1, lymphotoxin and tumour necrosis factor and evidence is accumulating that lymphotoxin is the major factor. Interleukin-6 is a growth factor for myeloma cells which is increased in patients with myeloma.

Investigations of hypercalcaemia in myeloma

Abnormal plasma proteins may bind to calcium increasing total serum calcium concentration which may be misleading as the free or ionised calcium level may be normal. True hypercalcaemia may be firmly diagnosed by a measurement of ionised calcium. Serum alkaline phosphatase is usually normal and it has been stated that the clinical combination of hypercalcaemia, normal alkaline phosphatase and renal impairment is caused by myeloma until proven otherwise.

Treatment of hypercalcaemia in myeloma

The treatment of malignant hypercalcaemia will be dealt with in detail but some special points about myeloma are noted. Renal impairment, caused by a possible combination of Bence–Jones proteinuria, hypercalcaemia, urinary tract infection and amyloidosis, is very common. Vigorous rehydration should be avoided in myeloma as left ventricular failure may be precipitated. Mithramycin should be avoided as it is nephrotoxic. The choice of treatment now falls between oral prednisolone, subcutaneous calcitonin and oral or parenteral bisphosphonates, or combination of these drugs depending on response.

Hypercalcaemia in non-myelomatous haematological malignancies

Hypercalcaemia may occasionally occur in T-cell lymphomas and rarely in B-cell lymphomas and histiocytic lymphomas. Bone lesions are frequent in Burkitt's lymphoma. It is possible that increased synthesis of 1,25 dihydroxyvitamin D may play a part in the hypercalcaemia of some lymphomas. Hypercalcaemia is very common in patients with adult T-cell leukaemia. It is likely that, as more patients with AIDS develop myeloproliferative disease, hypercalcaemia will become more common in this group.

Hypercalcaemia rarely occurs in Hodgkin's disease, chronic lymphocytic leukaemia and acute leukaemia.

The treatment of malignant hypercalcaemia (Table 5.8)

Hypercalcaemia is the cause of many unpleasant symptoms (see above) and its development is a near terminal event. The doctor is therefore not able to cure his patient but, equally, his objective should be that no patient dies

Table. 5.8. *Available therapy for malignant hypercalcaemia*

---

1. Tumour ablation
2. Rehydration
3. Loop diuretics, e.g. frusemide
4. Bisphosphonates
5. Calcitonin
6. Glucocorticoids
7. Mithramycin (plicamycin)
8. Phosphate
9. Prostaglandin synthetase inhibitors, e.g. indomethacin

---

with hypercalcaemia. In most patients, hypercalcaemia is caused by a combination of increased bone resorption and reduced renal calcium excretion. Clearly, the ideal would be to remove or ablate the tumour responsible and a specialist in radiotherapy and oncology should always be consulted to advise on the appropriate use of his specific tools. A discussion of radiotherapy and chemotherapy is outside the range of this book.

Most patients present with serum calcium less than 3.5 mmol/l and so treatment is usually not an urgent requirement and there is time for well-directed assessments and investigations. Patients with serum calcium of more than 3.5 mmol/l require more urgent attention. These figures are not absolute guides and clearly the general condition of the patient will help to determine management.

Maintenance treatment (serum calcium less than 3.5 mmol/l)

The choice of treatment falls between the following which may be used alone or in combination:

1. oral bisphosphonates
2. oral phosphate
3. oral prednisolone
4. subcutaneous calcitonin
5. mithramycin (plicamycin)
6. indomethacin

Bisphosphonates

Bisphosphonates are stable analogues of pyrophosphate and are characterised by the substitution of a P-C-P backbone for the P-O-P of pyrophosphate. They bind to hydroxyapatite, thereby inhibiting mineralisation, but

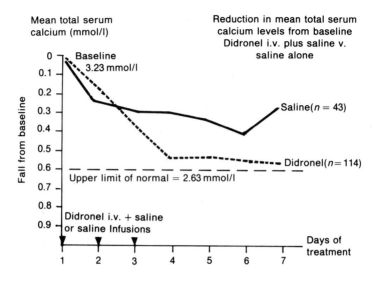

Fig. 5.5. The effect of intravenous etidronate (Didronel) on malignant hypercalcaemia.

their dominant effect in clinical practice is their ability to inhibit osteoclastic bone resorption.

Etidronate was the first compound introduced to clinical practice and has been used successfully in the treatment of Paget's disease, osteoporosis and malignant hypercalcaemia. Pamidronate (APD) and clodronate are later generation bisphosphonates which are now licensed for the treatment of malignant hypercalcaemia in the United Kingdom and Europe but not so far in the USA.

Bisphosphonates probably inhibit the development of osteoclasts and also probably have a direct effect on mature osteoclasts. Different compounds have variable capacities to inhibit mineralisation. Etidronate is the most likely to do this but this point is probably irrelevant in the discussion of a terminal condition.

Etidronate–The oral dose is 5–10 mg/kg/day. Higher doses are more likely to impair mineralisation. It is administered intravenously in doses of 7.5 mg/kg/day for 7 days and is effective in at least 75% of patients (Fig. 5.5). Etidronate is not so effective in treating hypercalcaemia when used orally without preceding intravenous therapy (Fig. 5.6). This is difficult to understand as it is effective when used orally in Paget's disease. Oral etidronate may be used to maintain normocalcaemia after an intravenous course or may be used orally after intravenous pamidronate or clodronate.

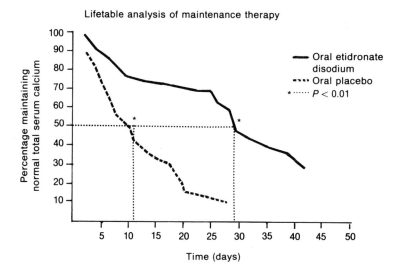

Fig. 5.6. The effect of oral etidronate (Didronel) on malignant hypercalcaemia. Note that oral etidronate is most appropriately used to help suppress hypercalcaemia after an intravenous course. (From Ringenberg & Rich, 1987.)

Pamidronate–Oral absorption is, as with all bisphosphonates, poor and the intravenous route is strongly favoured. Oral pamidronate is not at present available in the UK. Initial experience recommended the use of small doses of 15 mg/day for about 7 days or until normocalcaemia has been achieved, but single infusions of higher doses are now advocated. Many patients will respond for a worthwhile period to single infusions of 30–60 mg, but doses of up to 105 mg given over 24 hours have been given safely by the author. The infusion rate should not exceed 7.5–15 mg/hour, and the concentration in the infusion fluid should not exceed 15 mg/125 ml.

Pamidronate is very effective for 95% of patients with hypercalcaemia of malignancy or osteolytic bone disease, and it has a more rapid and more prolonged effect than etidronate or clodronate. Normocalcaemia is usually achieved within one week of single infusion, and maintained for several weeks depending on disease severity and chosen dose. Simultaneous use of calcitonin may give an even faster response.

Clodronate–This is available in the UK in both oral and intravenous forms. The oral dose is 0.8–3.2 g daily, but the intravenous route is probably preferable. One suitable regimen would be 300 mg in 0.5 litres of normal saline given over at least 2 hours daily for 5 days, but larger doses given as single infusions will be effective. There has been less experience with clodronate than pamidronate.

The toxicity of the bisphosphonates–Etidronate may impair bone mineralisation and increase serum phosphate by increasing renal tubular reabsorption. Pamidronate and clodronate do not impair mineralisation at the doses currently used. Pamidronate may cause transient fever and lymphopenia. Minor asymptomatic hypocalcaemia may also occur. No toxicity on other systems has yet been reported. An early report linking clodronate with leukaemia has not been confirmed.

Calcitonin

Calcitonin inhibits bone resorption by a direct action on the osteoclast and also by a less important effect on the kidney and the gut to increase calcium and phosphate excretion. Its use is limited by its temporary effect and by 'escape' from its action, presumably by upregulation of the calcitonin receptor rather than through a neutralising antibody effect.

Salmon calcitonin (salcatonin) is most widely used and can be given subcutaneously, intramuscularly or intravenously in doses of 50–200 units daily. Administration by nasal spray is a recent development and may increase the use of calcitonin in the maintenance of normocalcaemia. The dose is 50–400 units daily.

Calcitonin may cause nausea and vomiting as well as an unpleasant flushing sensation which may compel stopping therapy. An anti-emetic is helpful.

Calcitonin when used alone is usually only effective for 2–3 days and many patients are resistant to it. It is most effectively used in conjunction with prednisolone and can be combined with bisphosphonates as it has a more rapid action.

Oral phosphate

Oral phosphate reduces calcium absorption from the gut and also inhibits bone resorption. It is given as neutral sodium phosphate at 2–3 g/day in divided doses. Its use is limited by its major side-effect of diarrhoea and it may also predispose to renal stones, muscle pains and soft tissue calcification. Intravenous phosphate, once advocated, is dangerous and now always contraindicated when so many effective alternatives are available.

Glucocorticoids

Prednisolone 20–30 mg/day in divided doses is often effective in suppressing malignant hypercalcaemia and is probably the treatment of choice for maintaining normocalcaemia in patients with myeloma with or without a bisphosphonate. A consideration of late side-effects, e.g. osteoporosis, is less appropriate in this context. The mode of action is by inhibition of gut calcium uptake and probably by a direct anti-bone resorption mechanism.

Mithramycin (plicamycin)

Mithramycin is a cytotoxic drug with probably a direct action on osteoclasts. It is administered intravenously at 15–25 µg/kg/day for between 1 and 7 days depending on response. It is effective in 80% of patients and, before the advent of bisphosphonates, was probably the single most useful drug for the treatment of malignant hypercalcaemia. Its toxicity to liver, kidney, and bone marrow limits its use, and it is contraindicated in patients with renal impairment and in myeloma. Daily monitoring of marrow, liver and renal function is essential.

Prostaglandin inhibitors

Only about 10% of patients respond to indomethacin but it can be useful as a symptomatic treatment for malignant bone pain while helping to suppress hypercalcaemia in conjunction with other agents.

Emergency treatment for malignant hypercalcaemia

This is indicated for patients suffering significant hypercalcaemic symptoms or who have a serum calcium more than 3.5 mmol/l. Patients with 'parathyroid crisis' (see p. 129) should be managed in this way although prednisolone will be ineffective. Any drugs which might be contributing to hypercalcaemia, e.g. thiazides, should be stopped. Treatment should comprise:

1. rehydration
2. intravenous bisphosphonate
3. calcitonin
4. oral (or parenteral) prednisolone

Rehydration

Severely hypercalcaemic patients are profoundly dehydrated by the renal failure to concentrate urine. Volume depletion leads to enhanced sodium and calcium reabsorption. Sodium repletion impairs renal tubular calcium reabsorption and leads to a calcium diuresis. Intravenous isotonic saline is the most appropriate fluid replacement. Severely ill patients may need central venous monitoring and intensive care facilities. Patients may be depleted of 5–10 litres of extra-cellular fluid, and a replacement of 3–4 litres in the first 24 hours is appropriate. This will often achieve normocalcaemia but the patient will rapidly relapse if specific therapy is not also administered. Occasionally hypernatraemia is caused by the use of isotonic saline which should then be replaced by 5% dextrose.

Frusemide has been widely used with rehydration to promote urinary sodium and calcium excretion. It is clearly potentially hazardous to use a powerful diuretic in patients who are severely dehydrated, and there is little evidence to support its use. It may be useful in the rare patient who is over-hydrated or in cardiac failure, but its use should be confined to patients in whom central venous pressure is being monitored.

Bisphosphonates

These are the drugs of choice to be combined with rehydration. Either etidronate 7.5 mg/kg/day given in 3 litres of isotonic saline, or pamidronate 60 mg given in 3 litres of isotonic saline as a single infusion over 24 hours is highly successful. Both drugs should be used cautiously in patients with renal impairment, but are probably entirely safe in patients who are being adequately rehydrated.

Calcitonin and glucocorticoids

These are safe in renal failure and this property gives an advantage in such patients. Salcatonin 200 units every 12 hours subcutaneously combined with hydrocortisone hemisuccinate 100 mg every 6 hours will successfully reduce serum calcium to an acceptable concentration in most patients. Subsequent doses can be tapered depending on daily measurements of serum calcium.

Dialysis

This is occasionally necessary for patients with severe hypercalcaemia who are in renal failure, e.g. myeloma, and when other therapies are contraindicated or ineffective.

Further reading

Mundy, G.R. (1990). *Calcium Homeostasis: Hypercalcaemia and Hypocalcaemia*. Martin Dunitz. 2nd edn, pp. 1–272.
Ringenberg, Q.S. & Rich, P.S. (1987). *Clinical Therapeutics*, **9**, 318–25.

6

The hypocalcaemic patient

Introduction

In this chapter, the major disorders associated with hypocalcaemia, including renal bone disease, are discussed except for osteomalacia which has its own chapter. Many acute disorders may cause apparent hypocalcaemia mainly on account of a low plasma albumin, and thus a low total serum calcium as just over 50% of the calcium is bound, mainly to plasma proteins, predominantly albumin, with a small fraction bound to inorganic salts. Thus it is the 48% of calcium in ionised form that is metabolically active. Parathyroid hormone secretion is generally controlled by ionised calcium levels and they are only rarely reduced in these circumstances. Diagnosis of hypocalcaemia can thus only be made either by measuring the ionised calcium or by applying a correction for plasma albumin, a formula commonly used is:

$$Ca_c = Ca_p + [(40 - Alb_p) \times 0.02].$$

where Ca_c = corrected calcium (mmol/l)

$\quad Ca_p$ = plasma calcium (mmol/l)

$\quad Alb_p$ = plasma albumin (g/l)

$\quad 40$ = mean plasma albumin (g/l) of population (this may vary according to methodology used to measure albumin)

Many laboratories perform this calculation automatically and give the corrected calcium. It is not valid for large variations from the mean albumin.

The acid–base status of the patient is also relevant as an acidosis will result in a higher proportion of ionised calcium for a given total serum calcium level. Similarly with an alkalosis there will be a lower ionised calcium level and thus a greater potential for the symptoms of hypocalcaemia to manifest themselves. Causes of hypocalcaemia can be divided

141

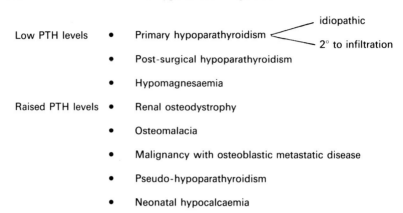

Fig. 6.1. Classification of hypocalcaemia.

into those which cause a compensatory rise in PTH levels and those which do not (Fig. 6.1). Measurement of parathyroid hormone (PTH) levels are, however, only necessary for the diagnosis of the rare forms of hypoparathyroidism.

Clinical manifestations of hypocalcaemia

A relatively rapid onset of the principal manifestations of hypocalcaemia are related to increased irritability of the neuromuscular system. Initially these present as parasthesiae and tingling periorally and in the extremities, followed by carpopedal spasm, laryngospasm with stridor (especially in children) and grand mal fits. Chovstek's sign (twitching of the corner of the mouth proceeding to contraction of all the ipsilateral facial muscles on tapping the facial nerve) may be present, as may Trousseau's sign (painful carpal spasm accompanied by parasthesiae after compression of the upper arm with a blood pressure cuff inflated above systolic pressure for 2 minutes). However, hyperventilation causing a respiratory alkalosis may give rise to these symptoms. The clinical situation and, if necessary, measurement of total serum calcium levels and blood gases will distinguish this from true hypocalcaemia. An acute fall in serum calcium may also cause a prolonged Q–T interval on an ECG and exacerbate cardiac failure.

Chronic hypocalcaemia of slow onset is often clinically asymptomatic. Rarely, it is associated with papilloedema. More commonly, calcification of the basal ganglia and cataracts occur owing to deposition of calcium phosphate salts. Chronic confusional states, which are reversible on correction of the hypocalcaemia, are also seen. The proximal myopathy often seen in osteomalacic states, however, is not usually associated with any of the other causes of hypocalcaemia.

The acute symptoms of hypocalcaemia depend upon its severity and the rate at which the calcium level has dropped. Thus the aggressiveness of the treatment will depend on clinical judgement. Acute symptoms, however will respond initially to 10 ml of 10% calcium gluconate infused over 10 minutes. 20–30 ml of 10% calcium gluconate diluted in 1 l of 0.9% saline run in 8 hourly is then usually sufficient to maintain normocalcaemia. The longer-term management will depend on the underlying cause and is discussed under the individual disorders.

Primary hypoparathyroidism

This rare typically auto-immune condition may occur at any age as an isolated finding or associated with other endocrine abnormalities, e.g. hypoadrenalism, hypothyroidism, diabetes mellitus and ovarian failure, any of which may follow by many years the initial isolated endocrine gland failure. It may also be associated with other manifestations of auto-immune disorders such as alopecia, vitiligo, pernicious anaemia or mucocutaneous candidiasis. Auto-antibodies are often found but they do not necessarily correlate with the gland affected. Very rarely, a familial form is seen which is associated with a failure of synthesis and/or secretion of PTH. Most cases present by young adulthood but some present later in life. Children are of normal height and build unlike those affected by pseudohypoparathyroidism.

Bone biochemistry in this condition consists of

(i)   hypocalcaemia 2^0 to lack of PTH giving rise to low bone resorption, low calcium reabsorption in the renal tubules and calcium malabsorption caused by low 1:25 hydroxyvitamin D levels.
(ii) Hyperphosphataemia because of increased renal tubular absorption.
(iii) Normal alkaline phosphatase.
Hypoparathyroidism is confirmed by unmeasurable PTH levels.

Treatment

As one of the major aetiological factors in hypocalcaemia is the failure of the conversion of 25-hydroxyvitamin D to 1:25-dihydroxyvitamin D due to lack of PTH, it is logical to treat hypoparathyroidism by either long-term calcitriol or alphacalcidol therapy 0.5–2.0 µg/d. These work by directly increasing calcium absorption from the gut as well as by appearing to have a direct effect on renal tubular reabsorption of calcium. The near physiological dosage regime of the hydroxylated metabolites is to be preferred to the large pharmacological doses of Vitamin D which were previously used. Similarly, as the hydroxylated metabolites are water soluble and therefore not stored in fat reserves (unlike the fat soluble Vitamin D), it is easier to achieve better control.

Calcium supplementation is preferable if there is any doubt about the sufficiency of calcium in the diet. The aim is to provide about 1 g of elemental calcium.

Post-surgical hypoparathyroidism

This is the most common form of hypoparathyroidism and can occur transiently following any operation on the anterior neck. Series post-partial thyroidectomy give an incidence of 1–4% for permanent hypoparathyroidism. The hypocalcaemia is often asymptomatic and does not require treatment. Normally the symptoms of hypocalcaemia present acutely within one week of the operation but the chronic state may develop many years following surgery, presumably secondary to the arterial supply becoming compromised during the operation.

The acute symptomatic post-operative condition is more likely to occur after removal of a parathyroid adenoma which has been associated with severe bone disease. Removal of the adenoma allows a 'hungry bones' syndrome to occur as the state of excessive resorption is replaced by rapid bone formation. Prolonged treatment may be required initially with calcium gluconate infusions followed by oral calcium supplements in addition to alphacalcidol or calcitriol in divided dosages of up to 4 µg/d. It is generally recommended that calcium supplements should be withdrawn prior to discharge from hospital as the combination of calcium supplements and a hydroxylated Vitamin D metabolite can easily result in severe hypercalcaemia. On discharge, the plasma calcium requires regular monitoring as the Vitamin D requirement will fall as the parathyroid function recovers and/or bone requirements reduce.

Magnesium deficiency

Magnesium deficiency is a condition associated with malabsorption syndrome, chronic parenteral nutrition and acute/chronic alcohol abuse. Drugs such as the aminoglycosides and cisplatin have also rarely been associated with hypomagnesaemia.

The hypocalcaemia seen in this condition is classically associated with severe hypokalaemia and only occurs when serum magnesium levels are very low (<0.4 mmol/l). PTH levels are often undetectable. The hypocalcaemia is caused by

(i) the parathyroid gland's requirement for Mg^{2+} in order to release PTH. (It is worth noting that this is the opposite effect to that of mild hypomagnesaemia which actually acts as a stimulus for PTH secretion.);
(ii) a peripheral block on the renal and skeletal actions of PTH which may take several days to return to normal.

Treatment consists of calcium supplements and initially i.v. magnesium salts, e.g. magnesium chloride 50 mmol in 1 l of 5% dextrose infused over 12–24 hrs. Oral magnesium preparations are poorly absorbed and often result in diarrhoea, but magnesium hydroxide probably causes the fewest side-effects.

Pseudohypoparathyroidism

This is a rare inherited disorder of tissue resistance to the effect of PTH. It usually presents before the age of 8 years and is more common in females. Typically, they have a classical appearance of short stature, round face with a short neck, short 4th and 5th metacarpals and subnormal intelligence. Band keratopathy (corneal calcification) and calcification of the basal ganglia are also seen. It was initially thought to be caused by absent or defective PTH receptors. This is now thought to be unlikely as the explanation for most cases and more recent studies suggest that there is an inhibitor of PTH in the plasma.

Biochemically they present as hypocalcaemia with hyperphosphataemia but have a raised PTH level in contrast to the low PTH levels found in patients with hypoparathyroidism. Both bone and kidneys are resistant to the action of PTH. A variant, known as **pseudopseudohypoparathyroidism**, can be found in the same families, in which the physical features are present but without the biochemical abnormalities. Treatment of pseudohypoparathyroidism is by the use of the hydroxylated metabolites but unfortunately only the biochemical abnormalities respond and the subnormal intelligence is unaffected by treatment.

Other causes

DeGeorges syndrome is a rare congenital form of hypoparathyroidism associated with failure of development of organs derived from the third and

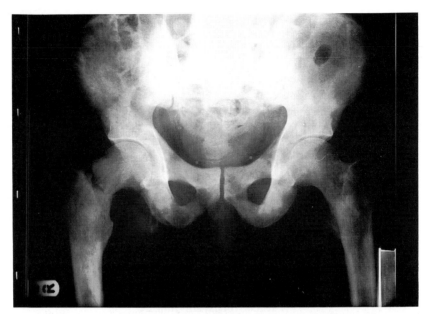

Fig. 6.2. X-ray of pelvis of man with multiple bony secondaries from a carcinoma of the prostate. (Reproduced by kind permission of Dr D.B. Evans.)

fourth branchial pouches. The thymus and the parathyroid glands are absent and the condition is fatal in early infancy.

Infiltration of the parathyroid glands by metastatic carcinoma or by heavy metal accumulation, e.g. copper in Wilson's Disease or iron in thalassaemia or haemochromatosis has been described.

True hypocalcaemia is also seen in **acute pancreatitis** and is probably multifactorial in origin. Impaired PTH secretion in response to the hypocalcaemic stimulus has been noted in some studies as well as the usually accepted explanation of calcium sequestration by the fatty acids released by fat necrosis.

Chelation of ionised calcium by **citrated blood** transfused rapidly in large amounts can cause rapid falls in calcium and it should be customary in those circumstances to routinely give 10 ml of 10% calcium gluconate after 8 units, repeating it again as necessary.

Rarely **sclerotic bone metastases** (Fig. 6.2), e.g. prostatic or breast cancer can cause hypocalcaemia due to the excessive osteoblastic stimulation exceeding the capacity of the parathyroid gland to respond.

Treating severe osteomalacia with Vitamin D without calcium supplements can cause worsening of the hypocalcaemia on account of the sudden uptake of available calcium, the **'hungry bones' syndrome**.

Neonatal hypocalcaemia is commonly seen and can be divided into an early form occurring in the first 24 h of life and a late form, usually occurring after the first week of life. The early form characteristically is seen in premature and sick infants. The cause is unknown but it does not appear to be due to immature parathyroid glands or abnormal Vitamin D metabolism. It has been postulated that the sudden withdrawal of the placental calcium supply at a time of maximum need overwhelms the homeostatic mechanism. Late hypocalcaemia can occur in infants born to hyperparathyroid mothers where the maternal hypercalcaemia causes a normally transient suppression of the infants parathyroid function. It is also found in infants fed on cows' milk formula feeds containing high phosphate concentrations.

Renal bone disease

Introduction

The kidneys play a central role in bone metabolism by

(i)   maintaining calcium and phosphate balance via the renal tubules;
(ii) activating Vitamin D to 1,25 D by the action of 1 α-hydroxylase;
(iii) allowing excretion of potentially osteotoxic substances, e.g. aluminium;
(iv) degrading and excreting PTH.

Renal osteodystrophy (Fig. 6.3) is predominantly associated with two forms of bone disease, osteitis fibrosa and osteomalacia. In addition osteosclerosis, osteoporosis and growth retardation are seen.

Osteitis fibrosa is the bone disease associated with raised parathyroid hormone (PTH) levels. Hyperparathyroidism is usually the earliest manifestation of renal bone disease with minor histological changes being detected in the majority of patients with glomerular filtration rates of less than 60 ml/min, although only a few will be clinically symptomatic. The hyperparathyroidism is caused by

(i)   hypocalcaemia due to (a) the direct effect of phosphate retention on the $Ca \times PO_4$ product (b) decreased 1:25-dihydroxyvitamin D production caused by renal tissue damage and the effect or raised phosphate levels on 1-α hydroxylase activity (c) skeletal resistance to the action of PTH
(ii) reduced degradation and excretion of PTH by the kidneys.
(iii) the parathyroid glands appearing to require higher ionized calcium levels to suppress PTH production than in non uraemic controls.

Osteomalacia is principally caused by low levels of 1,25-dihyd-

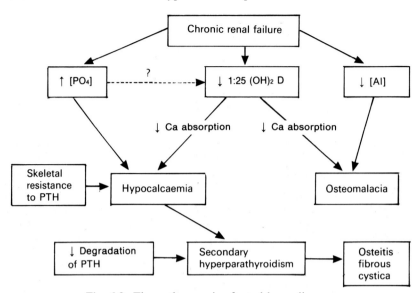

Fig. 6.3. The pathogenesis of renal bone disease.

roxyvitamin D and the retention of aluminium. 1,25-dihydroxyvitamin D
levels only significantly drop in severe renal failure (GFR ‹30 ml/min) and
studies suggest that the prevalence of histological osteomalacia in patients
with end-stage renal failure is between 25 and 30%. **Adynamic osteomalacia**
is most commonly associated with patients on maintenance dialysis (on
account of aluminium accumulation associated with the dialysis fluid and
the use of phosphate binders). However, it has rarely been a clinical
problem in adults prior to dialysis therapy being commenced and now that
aluminium binders are rarely used and dialysate fluids strictly controlled by
the manufacturers, it is now rare even in the dialysis population.
Osteoporosis and **osteosclerosis** often coexist and are common in chronic
renal failure. Cortical thinning is the initial feature of osteoporosis and is
seen even in mild renal disease and is probably associated with early
compensated secondary hyperparathyroidism. Other possible aetiological
factors include lack of dietary calcium and protein, hypogonadism, steroid
treatment for the underlying renal disease and the use of heparin during
renal dialysis. Osteosclerosis is observed in some patients by the X-ray
changes seen in the vertebrae known as 'rugger jersey spine.' (Fig. 6.4)

Clinical features

The majority of the clinical manifestations of renal osteodystrophy tend to
present late and are associated with the musculo-skeletal system. *Bone pain,*

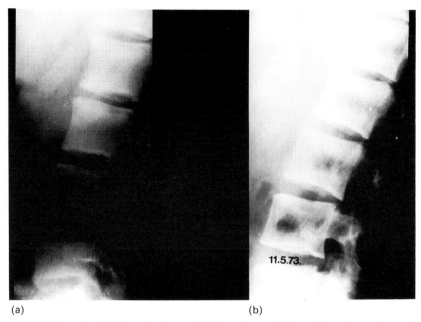

(a)   (b)

Fig. 6.4. Vertebral bodies of patient with chronic renal failure (*a*) at diagnosis, and (*b*) 4 years later showing the development of a 'rugger jersey spine' appearance. (Reproduced by kind permission of Dr D.B. Evans.)

however, may be an early feature and is usually rather vague and diffuse in nature, most common in the lower back, pelvis and legs. A *proximal myopathy* may rarely be present. Both of these symptoms, classically associated with osteomalacia, can occur even when the predominant bone lesion is osteitis fibrosa. *Fractures* may occur in osteitis fibrosa, but are particularly associated with aluminium osteomalacia. *Acute arthritis* (pseudogout) can also occur, often associated with periarticular calcification caused by accumulation of hydroxyapatite crystals. Vascular calcification is also common. Other rarer *extraosseous manifestations* usually associated with metastatic calcification include pulmonary involvement and red eyes (conjunctival calcification). *Pruritus* in renal failure is multi-factorial in origin but one of the mechanisms implicated is deposition of calcium in the skin. Some patients with both severe arterial calcification and secondary hyperparathyroidism may develop on *acute ischaemic necrosis* of the tips of the fingers and toes (calciphylaxis). A cardiomyopathy has been described associated with high PTH levels. *Skeletal deformities* can occur in adults with longstanding disease as well as in children. In the latter, genu valgum and bowed tibiae and femora are not uncommon, whereas in adults the most common abnormalities are ribcage deformities, lumbar scoliosis and thoracic kyphosis. *Growth regardation* is also noted in children secondary to malnutrition, renal bone disease and chronic acidosis in spite of growth hormone levels usually being very high. Aluminium associated bone disease is characterised by severe bone pain and fractures.

Biochemical features

In the initial stages of the disease plasma calcium levels are maintained by elevated PTH levels, but by the time GFR has fallen to < 30 ml/min, ionised calcium levels have started to drop due to an increase in the complexed fraction of plasma calcium. This is followed in advanced renal failure by true hypocalcaemia especially if there is underlying osteomalacia or a severe metabolic acidosis. Hypercalcaemia can also be encountered especially in dialysis patients taking calcium carbonate or receiving calcitriol therapy. Mild hypercalcaemia may also be a feature of aluminium bone disease.

Hyperphosphataemia occurs early in the uraemic patient but is not helpful in determining the presence of bone disease. Evidence suggests, however, that phosphate retention by producing a fall in ionised calcium, plays an important role in the production of secondary hyper-parathyroidism. There is little evidence for a direct effect.

Alkaline phosphatase levels, if raised, usually indicate underlying bone disease and levels correlate well with severity as well as being a helpful marker of response to treatment. They do not distinguish osteomalacia from osteitis fibrosa. There may be coexistent liver disease and alkaline phosphatase isoenzymes or gamma glutamyl transpeptidase estimations should be carried out to confirm that the raised levels are of bony origin. In dialysis osteomalacia, however, alkaline phosphatase as well as calcium levels may be normal and thus normal bone biochemistry does not rule out renal osteodystrophy.

Aluminium levels > 7.5 µmol/l are nearly always associated with bone toxicity.

PTH levels are apparently raised even in early renal failure, but it is important to ascertain that the assay used only measures the biologically active amino terminal fragment of the molecule. This is because, in renal failure, the biologically inactive carboxyl terminal fragment will accumulate and will not reflect parathyroid gland activity.

Radiological features

The earliest radiological features are of secondary hyperparathyroidism resulting in increased bone resorption, classically producing sub-periosteal

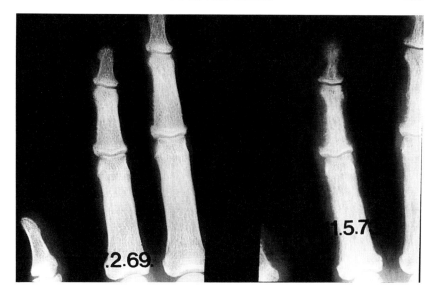

Fig. 6.5. Phalanges of patient with chronic renal failure (*a*) at diagnosis, and (*b*) 4 years later showing the development of subperiosteal erosions. (Reproduced by kind permission of Dr D.B. Evans.)

erosions and cysts of the terminal phalanges (Fig. 6.5), although other sites can be involved including the femoral and humeral necks, the proximal end of the tibia, the sacro-iliac joints and the ends of the clavicles. These signs correlate well with the histological features of osteitis fibrosa seen on bone biopsy. In addition, endosternal resorption takes place reducing the cortical width of long bones. In mainly trabecular bones, e.g. vertebral bodies hyperparathyroidism may stimulate new bone formation resulting in osteosclerosis giving rise to the typical 'rugger jersey' appearance (Fig. 6.3). Osteomalacic features may also be seen but unless a Looser's zone (which is pathognomonic of the disease) is present, the changes are non-specific and thus a bone biopsy needs to be performed in order to exclude this condition.

Extra-skeletal calcification can also take place on account of dystrophic calcium deposition and/or the raised calcium phosphate product. The most common abnormality is arterial calcification, although periarticular calcification giving rise to palpable masses can occur.

Radionuclide scanning

Technetium-labelled diphosphonate bone scans can be used to assess the severity of the bone disease as well as detecting pseudo-fractures and detecting response to treatment. However, they can only rarely be of use in determining the type of bone disease present and a bone biopsy is needed to distinguish osteitis fibrosa from osteomalacia. The scanning changes seen in osteitis fibrosa are those of the increase bone turnover due to raised PTH levels, i.e. a symmetrical increase in activity over the skull, sternum, vertebrae and distal aspects of the femur and tibia.

Histology

Bone biopsy is required to identify the type of bone disease present and to quantitate the aluminium content. In most cases, varying degrees of osteitis fibrosa and osteomalacic changes will coexist. In osteitis fibrosa, the increased turnover rate is illustrated by a large increase in the number of osteoblasts and osteoclasts as well as peritrabecular fibrosis. It was this hypercellularity that gave rise to the term 'osteitis' as they were initially thought to be inflammatory cells. In addition, the trabecular surface covered by osteoid and the osteoid volume will be increased but the mineralisation fronts are normal and osteoid seam thickness is not increased. Osteomalacia secondary to lack of 1,25-dihydroxyvitamin D or aluminium accumulation shows the classical changes of increased osteoid thickness and trabecular surface covered by osteoid as well as decreased mineralisation rate.

The patients with 'pure' osteomalacic changes are usually on dialysis and exhibit low turnover or 'aplastic' bone disease, usually associated with marked aluminium deposition although iron retention has also been implicated. They do not usually show evidence of secondary hyper-parathyroidism. This form of osteomalacia does not respond to 1,25-dihydroxyvitamin D therapy. In this state, osteoid volume is normal but there are few osteoblasts or osteoclasts and there is substantially reduced bone formation as measured by double tetracycline labelling. In this technique, tetracycline labelling is carried out twice, usually a fortnight apart resulting in two bands fluorescing under UV light on the bone biopsy. The rate of bone formation can thus be calculated from knowledge of the separation of the two bands as well as the length of bone surface covered.

Treatment

This aims to

(i)   control serum phosphate levels
(ii) replace Vitamin D

(iii) reduce PTH levels
(iv) reduce aluminium overload
(v) provide adequate calcium intake

Diet

The principal aim is to control the phosphate retention which is a major cause of secondary hyperparathyroidism and extra-skeletal calcification. Dietary phosphorus reduction from the average Western diet levels of 1.0–1.8 g/d to the ideal 400–800 g/d can be achieved by restriction of diary products and a low protein diet. Such diets, however, although effective in reducing PTH levels, are unpalatable with poor patient compliance and thus phosphate binders are usually given.

Calcium supplements are necessary as calcium absorption is decreased in uraemic patients and there is evidence that long term treatment with supplements in the order of 1 g/day reduces bone resorption and fracture incidence. In addition, calcium carbonate can act as a phosphate binding agent.

Phosphate binders

Aluminium hydroxide and aluminium carbonate have been used for many years to reduce intestinal phosphate absorption in patients on dialysis. They were considered unabsorbable, but it is now realised that aluminium can be absorbed resulting in aluminium induced bone disease as well as dialysis dementia. Calcium carbonate is now therefore generally used in doses varying between 4 and 12 g/d given in divided doses meals in order to maximise efficacy, dosages varying according to the approximate amount of phosphorus in each meal. Unfortunately, it may give rise to diarrhoea and it is not always effective in controlling hyperphosphataemia and thus aluminium hydroxide may still be required. Hypercalcaemia is the major side-effect and there is a possibility that long-term use will produce extra skeletal calcification. It is also on account of the risk of extra-skeletal calcification that calcium carbonate should not be given to patients with markedly raised phosphate levels unless the ionised calcium level is low. Hypercalcaemia is often a problem and patients may need to be dialysed against a very low calcium dialysate (1–1.25 mmol/l)

Vitamin D metabolites

Vitamin D supplementation is often used early in the disease in combination with diet, and the use of phosphate binding agents, in order to attempt to prevent the development of severe secondary hyperparathyroidism and osteitis fibrosa. Although other metabolites, e.g. 25-hydroxyvitamin D have been used in the USA, calcitriol (1,25-hydroxyvitamin D) or alfacalcidol (1-α hydroxyvitamin D) are usually used with dosages in the range of 0.25–1.5 μg/d. Studies show rapid symptomatic, biochemical and histological improvement of osteitis fibrosa. As healing occurs, the dose of Vitamin D required decreases. The major side-effect is hypercalcaemia which may present early in aluminium-related bone disease or after several months in patients with osteitis fibrosa responding to treatment. In the latter case, a drop in alkaline phosphatase levels to normal may herald the rise in serum calcium.

Chelation of aluminium

Aluminium is taken up by many tissues including bone and parathyroid tissue. Aluminium sulphate is added to water during purification as a flocculent as it helps to precipitate out organic matter. Concentrations of between 5 and 30 μmol/l are as a consequence found in drinking water. Water purification systems have been extensively used to reduce aluminium contamination of the dialysis fluids and aluminium levels are now strictly controlled by the manufacturers. Up to the recent past it was difficult to sufficiently reduce the aluminium concentration. In these cases, desferrioxamine was given, usually intravenously, which complexes with the protein-bound aluminium forming an ultrafiltrable compound which can be removed by the kidneys or dialysis. Side-effects include allergic skin reactions, anaphlaxis and general malaise. Regular ophthalmic review is required as, probably on account of chelation of other trace minerals, optic neuropathy and maculopathy can occur.

Parathyroidectomy

This is indicated when, despite the above treatment regimes, severe secondary hyperparathyroidism persists. Aluminium-related bone disease also must be excluded. The indicators include persistent hypercalcaemia, pruritis unresponsive to treatment, progressive extra-skeletal calcification and the appearance of severe ischaemic ulcers and necrosis (calciphylaxis).

Post-transplantation bone disease

After renal transplantation 1,25-dihydroxyvitamin D synthesis occurs and the osteomalacic component of the renal osteodystrophy usually heals within a year. Similarly, both ostitis fibrosa and aluminium related disease will heal if renal function remains satisfactory. However, hypercalcaemia and hypophosphataemia may occur due to pre-existing hyper-parathyroidism, with a peak incidence about six months post-transplantation. Hypophosphataemia post-transplantation is not solely due to hyperparathyroidism and both decreased intestinal phosphate absorption and the effect of corticosteroid therapy have been postulated. It was assumed that the hypophosphataemia would give rise to *osteomalacia* which was assumed to be a major cause of the fracturing bone disease seen post-transplantation, but more recent studies have failed to discover an increased incidence of the disease. *Avascular necrosis* has been the most common bony disorder on account of the use of high dose steroids for immunosuppression, with uncontrolled secondary hyperparathyroidism also being implicated in its aetiology. This condition presents with pain in the weight-bearing joints, especially the head of femur and humerus and the knees. These symptoms may occur prior to the development of radiological changes. However, with the advent of cyclosporin and a low dose corticosteroid immunosuppressive regime, the incidence is falling. *Osteoporosis* is also seen mainly on account of the long-term use of corticosteroids.

Further reading

Tzamaloukas, A.H. (1990). Diagnosis and management of bone disorders in chronic renal failure and dialyzed patients. In *The Medical Clinics of North America*, vol. 74(4) eds. Mandal, A.K. & Hebert, L.A.

Slatopolsky, E., Coburn, J.W. (1990). Renal osteodystrophy. In *Metabolic Bone Disease and Clinically Related Disorders* (2nd edn.) eds. Avioli, L.V. & Krane, S.M. W.B. Saunders Company, pp. 452–474.

Bilezikian, J.P. (1987). Clinical disorders of the parathyroid glands. In *Clinical Endocrinology of Calcium Metabolism* eds. Martin, T.J. & Raisz, L.G. Marcel Dekker Inc., New York, pp. 97–140.

7

Rarer bone disorders presenting as fractures

The rarer causes of pathological fractures

A summary of the differential diagnosis of pathological fractures is given in Fig. 7.1.

Patients presenting with a pathological fracture, i.e. a fracture resulting from no or minimal trauma can, in most cases, be easily diagnosed either from the X-ray appearances or from simple investigation of generalised osteopoenia described in Chapter 2. The purpose of this chapter is to provide background information on various rare forms of bone disease, although the investigation and care of such patients would normally be carried out by a specialised bone clinic.

Polyostotic fibrous dysplasia

This rare non-familial disorder may present at any age in males and females with fractures associated with cyst-like lesions in the cortex of any bones including the skull. Other lesions consist of expansions of the cortex with a 'ground glass' appearance. They are caused by the proliferation of osteoclasts and vascular fibrous tissue. They are often associated with skin pigmentation and if associated with precocious puberty (nearly always in females) comprises Albright's syndrome. It may be asymptomatic or present as an expansion of the bone cortex. Most lesions develop in early childhood and usually remain static in adult life. The differential diagnosis of such cysts is hyperparathyroidism. Treatment is supportive only.

Osteogenesis imperfecta

This is a group of hereditary disorders associated with abnormal collagen synthesis and composition. Although rare, it is the most common inherited

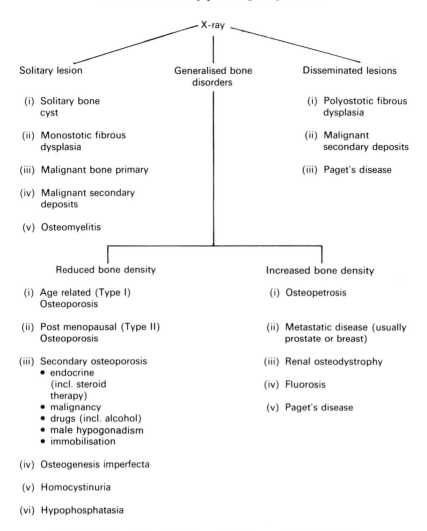

Fig. 7.1. The differential diagnosis of the pathological fracture

bone disorder with an estimated incidence in childhood of between 1:20000 and 1:60000 live births. The underlying disorder appears to consist of various mutations involving the gene concerned with the production of Type I collagen in bone. The collagen fibres may be reduced in size, and bundle formation may be defective, or there may be diminished production of normal fibres. Classification of osteogenesis imperfecta (OI) is difficult as it is both genetically and clinically heterogeneous with both quantitative and qualitative variation within each genetic phenotype. The condition

Table. 7.1. *Modified Sillence classification of osteogenesis imperfecta.*

Type	Phenotype	Pattern of Inheritance
I	Mild OI, relatively few fractures, non-deforming mild scoliosis. Blue sclerae, adult hearing loss. Dentinogenesis imperfecta (Type IB) in 25%.	AD
IIA	Lethal OI, Multiple intra-uterine fractures, broad short femora, continous beading of ribs, defective mineralisation of the calvarium.	AD: new mutations
IIB	As IIA, except that ribs are thin, with or without continuous beading, and the calvarium is better mineralised.	AR
IC	Less frequent than type A or B. Femora and humeri are longer, undermodelled, and irregular. Calvarium is poorly mineralised.	AR (data limited)
III	Severe OI with frequent fracture rate and marked deformity. Marked growth retardation. Scoliosis severe and may progress to compromised pulmonary function. White or blue sclerae.	AD (75%) AR (25%)
IV	Moderately severe disease. Heterogenous phenotype, white or blue sclerae. Fractures may be frequent and are asssociated with obvious skeletal deformity. Scoliosis is moderately severe. Dentinogenesis imperfecta (Type IVB) in 25%, adult hearing loss.	AD

Key: AD: autosomal dominant; AR: autosomal recessive
* Modified from Sillence DO Osteogenesis imperfecta: nosology and genetics. Ann. NY Acad. Sci. **543**, 1–15, (1988).
(Reproduced by permission from Avioli & Krane *Metabolic Bone Disease* 2nd ed.).

however is characterised by osteoporosis, brittle bones, joint laxity, blue sclerae, deafness, dental deformities and thin skin. There are several new classifications which divide the various forms of the condition according to the clinical classification and mode of inheritance but even then there may be difficulty in classifying an individual patient. A modification of Sillence's classification which associates clinical phenotypes with pattern of inheritance is given in Table 7.1, but a detailed account is out of the scope of this book. The traditional classification divides the disease into two main groupings according to age of onset and severity.

(i) 'Osteogenesis imperfecta congenita' or lethal osteogenesis imperfecta (Fig. 7.2) presents in utero or in the neonatal period and may be the result

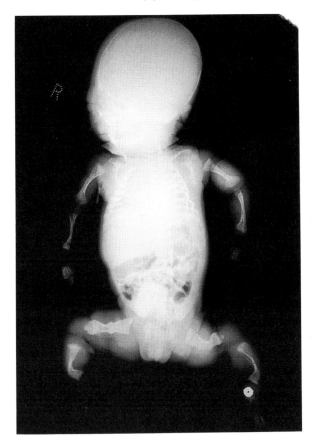

Fig. 7.2. X-ray of stillborn foetus with lethal Type II osteogenesis imperfecta showing multiple fractures and deformities of the lower limbs. (Reproduced by kind permission of Dr J. Tudor.)

of a new mutation or with an autosomal dominant or recessive inheritance. They are all included in the Sillence-Type II classification. It is lethal on account of the multiple fractures and pulmonary insufficiency. In addition, the infants have a large head, thin calvarium, blue sclerae and deformed, short limbs. It is estimated that about 10% of cases of OI are of this type and about 25% are stillborn.

(ii) 'Osteogenesis imperfecta tarda' may present in the first year of life or later childhood. It embraces the Sillence-Types III, IV and I (listed in descending order of severity), now biochemically characterised by different type I collagen abnormalities. They predominantly have an autosomal dominant inheritance. In Type III and IV, fractures are usually present at birth. Both long bones and vertebrae may fracture resulting in scoliosis. In addition severe deformity occurs on account of microfractures in the more severe 'progressively deforming' Type III disease. Such patients often suffer between 20 and 30 fractures in childhood and usually rapidly become wheelchair bound. Severe growth retardation also occurs. Blue sclerae are common and brittle poorly aligned teeth (dentogenesis imperfecta) may be seen. Progressive adult hearing loss may occur. Types III and IV are

estimated to make up approximately 20% and 6% of cases, respectively. Type IV is termed moderately severe disease and is characterised by blue sclerae in infancy which fade with age. It is intermediate in severity between Types III and I.

Type I disease is the most common form of the disease affecting approximately 55–60% of sufferers, although the incidence may be higher as the diagnosis can easily be missed in less severe cases. It has an autosomal dominant inheritance, although it has been suggested that up to 30% are new mutations. The collagen molecules in these patients are qualitatively normal unlike the collagen found in the other forms of the disease and the abnormality appears to be a failure in production by the fibroblast. Patients in this group are only mildly affected with normal fracture healing and thus have no skeletal deformity. Although they exhibit radiological osteopoenia from birth, fractures usually affecting the lower limbs predominantly only occur when the child starts walking and fracture incidence shows a marked drop after puberty. Fractures at birth are uncommon. Joint laxity, mild growth retardation and deafness are common and the majority have blue sclera.

The differential diagnosis in children includes the 'battered baby' syndrome, homocystinuria, juvenile osteoprosis and malabsorption syndromes. In adults, the differential diagnosis of osteoporosis has to be considered. There are no specific biochemical markers of the disease although alkaline phosphatase may be raised on account of a recent fracture.

Although numerous agents have been tried, there is no effective medical therapy for this condition. There is no evidence of a mineralisation defect and thus Vitamin D therapy is ineffective. There is no evidence that Vitamin C intake has any effect. Aggressive surgical therapy correcting deformity usually by a rodding procedure is used to maintain function. Intensive rehabilitation including the use of braces as well as psychological support is also necessary.

Homocystinuria

This is an autosomal recessively inherited inborn error of methionine metabolism. This results in accumulation of homocysteine. Osteoporosis is seen particularly of the vertebrae; in addition, long bone fractures occur which are slow to heal. Patients have a Marfanoid appearance. Pyridoxine therapy has been reported to reverse the biochemical abnormalities in some patients.

Hypophosphatasia

The rare genetic defect resulting in defective alkaline phosphatase synthesis usually presents in infants but is increasingly being recognised in adults. It probably has an autosomal dominant form of inheritance in most cases and is characterised by reduction of alkaline phosphatase levels in serum, bone, kidneys and liver. Plasma and urine levels of an amino acid, phosphorylethanolamine, and pyrophosphate levels are raised. The effect of the deficiency in bone results in a mineralisation defect. The condition in children resembles very severe rickets with multiple fractures, although there is no known abnormality of Vitamin D metabolism. In addition, there is raised intracranial pressure and hypocalcaemia and in the homozygous form the condition is usually fatal in infancy. In the heterozygous form, the condition may present in adult life with growth retardation associated with osteopoenia, multiple fractures, early loss of secondary dentition and atypical osteomalacia. The biochemical findings are the same as in children and there is no effective treatment.

Conditions associated with generalised sclerosis

Osteopetrosis (Marble bone disease/Albers–Schonberg disease)

This is a rare disorder, usually of autosomal dominant (benign type) or autosomal recessive inheritance (malignant type) inheritance. It may present with a wide spectrum of severity varying from a chance radiological finding of bone sclerosis in adults with the benign disease to multiple pathological fractures and cranial nerve palsies. In addition, marrow cavities fail to develop leading to extramedullary haematopoiesis with hypersplenism, anaemia, decreased resistance to infection, and a fatal outcome in childhood. Adult disease is usually mild with excellent long-term survival and many patients are asymptomatic. Serum calcium and alkaline phosphatase levels are usually normal.

Radiologically the changes show in spectrum of changes from mild osteosclerosis often only seen in the vertebrae to the 'bone within bone'

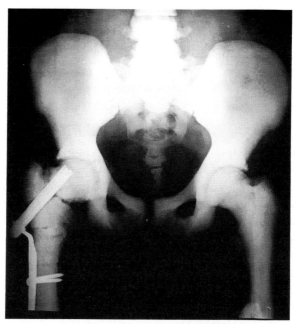

Fig. 7.3. X-ray of pelvis in patient with osteopetrosis. (Reproduced by kind permission of Dr J. Tudor.)

appearance in vertebral bodies which is diagnostic of the condition and generalised osteosclerosis with abnormal skeletal growth. Pathological fractures of long bones are often seen (Fig. 7.3).

The underlying pathological deficit appears to involve a failure of bone resorption on account of defective osteoclast function. Studies in mice with osteopetrosis have suggested that the underlying abnormality may be defective production of macrophage colony stimulating factor (M-CSF) by the osteoblast. M-CSF is a growth factor which has been shown to stimulate the formation of osteoclast-like cells. However, increased M-CSF levels have not been found in humans with the condition, and other studies have suggested a viral aetiology. Resistance to 1,25-dihydroxyvitamin D has also been suggested, as elevated levels of 1,25-dihydroxyvitamin D have been found in some patients and 1,25-dihydroxyvitamin D is involved in osteoclast formation. Histology of the affected bone in the benign form of the disease usually show a lack of osteoclasts and those which are present are abnormal. In the malignant form, the narrow spaces may be filled with fibrous tissue.

Characteristically, 'islands' of cartilage within bone trabecula are seen.

The treatment for the adult form of the disease is supportive but the malignant form in childhood has been treated with a calcium depleted diet and large doses of calcitriol in order to stimulate osteoclastic activity. Allogenic bone marrow transplantation has also been successfully carried out. Large doses of glucocorticoids have been used to combat the systemic effects.

Fluorosis

Probably the most common cause of fluorosis is associated with the use of sodium fluoride in the treatment of osteoporotic bone disease. It is, however, endemic in some areas of India, the Middle East and South Africa on account of contaminated well water, and has been seen as an occupational disease in the aluminium, steel and glass industry working with fluoride containing ores.

The bone manifestations include mottling of the teeth with pits in the enamel, generalised skeletal pain, arthropathy and stiffness especially in the back. Pain associated with stress fractures may also be seen. Fluoride produces osteosclerosis by direct stimulation of osteoblasts and the formation of fluoroapatite crystals which are more resistant to osteoclastic activity. This resistance to osteoclastic activity results in a tendency towards a lower ionised calcium level with resulting compensatory secondary hyperparathyroidism.

The radiological changes may be absent but there may be generalised osteosclerotic changes particularly seen in the vertebra with ligamental calcification especially around the pelvis. Osteomalacic changes are manifested by stress fractures.

Calcium and phosphate levels are usually normal but alkaline phosphatase levels may be raised on account of osteoblastic stimulation which also results in calcium retention.

Treatment is by reducing fluoride intake and giving calcium and Vitamin D if osteomalacic changes are found on bone biopsy.

Further reading

Beighton, P. (1988). *Inherited Disorders of the Skeleton.* 2nd edn. Churchill Livingstone, Edinburgh.

Rowe, D.W. & Shapiro, J.R. (1990). Osteogenesis imperfecta. In *Metabolic Bone Disease and Clinically Related Disorders* 2nd edn. eds. Avioli, L.V. & Krane, S.M. W.B. Saunders Company, pp. 659–701.

Index

- metabolic bone disorders
- hypercalcemia
- hypocalcemia